1,000,000 Books

are available to read at

———◆———

www.ForgottenBooks.com

———◆———

Read online
Download PDF
Purchase in print

ISBN 978-1-397-32848-9
PIBN 11374261

This book is a reproduction of an important historical work. Forgotten Books uses
state-of-the-art technology to digitally reconstruct the work, preserving the original format
whilst repairing imperfections present in the aged copy. In rare cases, an imperfection in
the original, such as a blemish or missing page, may be replicated in our edition. We do,
however, repair the vast majority of imperfections successfully; any imperfections that
remain are intentionally left to preserve the state of such historical works.

Forgotten Books is a registered trademark of FB &c Ltd.
Copyright © 2018 FB &c Ltd.
FB &c Ltd, Dalton House, 60 Windsor Avenue, London, SW19 2RR.
Company number 08720141. Registered in England and Wales.

For support please visit www.forgottenbooks.com

1 MONTH OF
FREE
READING

at
www.ForgottenBooks.com

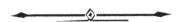

By purchasing this book you are eligible for one month membership to ForgottenBooks.com, giving you unlimited access to our entire collection of over 1,000,000 titles via our web site and mobile apps.

To claim your free month visit:

www.forgottenbooks.com/free1374261

* Offer is valid for 45 days from date of purchase. Terms and conditions apply.

English
Français
Deutsche
Italiano
Español
Português

www.forgottenbooks.com

Mythology Photography **Fiction**
Fishing Christianity **Art** Cooking
Essays Buddhism Freemasonry
Medicine **Biology** Music **Ancient
Egypt** Evolution Carpentry Physics
Dance Geology **Mathematics** Fitness
Shakespeare **Folklore** Yoga Marketing
Confidence Immortality Biographies
Poetry **Psychology** Witchcraft
Electronics Chemistry History **Law**
Accounting **Philosophy** Anthropology
Alchemy Drama Quantum Mechanics
Atheism Sexual Health **Ancient History**
Entrepreneurship Languages Sport
Paleontology Needlework Islam
Metaphysics Investment Archaeology
Parenting Statistics Criminology
Motivational

Vol. III.—No. 12.　　　　1st DECEMBER.　　　　1905

THE

OPHTHALMOSCOPE

A MONTHLY REVIEW OF CURRENT OPHTHALMOLOGY.

Editors:

SYDNEY STEPHENSON
(London).

CHARLES A. OLIVER
(Philadelphia).

Sub-Editor:

C. DEVEREUX MARSHALL
(London).

Correspondents:

Dr. JAMES BARRETT and Dr. T. K. HAMILTON (Australasia); Dr. P. COOTE (Canada); Major H. HERBERT (East Indies); Dr. C. MANCHÉ (Malta); Dr. FRANK W. MARLOW (United States of North America); Dr. A. DARIER (France); Dr. G. F. ROCHAT (Holland); Dr. A. BIRCH-HIRSCHFELD (Germany); Dr. RICKARD VIDÉKY (Austria-Hungary); Dr. A. ANTONELLI (Italy); Dr. H. COPPEZ (Belgium); Professor HAAB (Switzerland); Prof. WIDMARK (Scandinavia); Dr. EMILIO ALVARADO and Dr. ADOLFO ALVAREZ (Spain); and Dr. M. URIBE-TRONCOSO (Mexico).

PRICE ONE SHILLING.

(Annual Subscription 10/6 *Prepaid*.)

London:

GEORGE PULMAN AND SONS, LTD.,

24-26, Thayer Street, W.

1905.

Copyright.]　　　　　　　　　　　[Entered at Stationers' Hall.

URRY & PAXTON

Ophthalmic Opticians,

195, GREAT PORTLAND STREET

LONDON, W.

And at LIVERPOOL & BRISTOL.

CURRY & PAXTON are the only Optician who do *not* prescribe glasses, and who wor exclusively to Surgeons' prescriptions.

Provincial Surgeons are now enabled to prescrib properly fitted frames as well as correct lenses if they adop the system advocated by CURRY & PAXTON.

NOTE.—All Ophthalmic Instruments manufactured by the firm have the firm's name legibly engraved upon them. None genuine without the Name.

The Luminous Retinoscope.

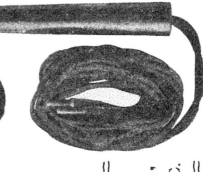

DE ZENG'S Luminous Ophthalmoscope

View of the Retina obtained with de Zeng Ophthalmoscope.

	£	s	d
De Zeng's Luminous Ophthalmoscope, Loring's	3	3	0
De Zeng's Luminous Retinoscope	3	3	0
Portable Batteries for same	1	1	0
De Zeng's ... thus Ophthalmoscope, model English Morton	9	7	6
De Zeng's ... thus Ophthalmoscope, model American Morton	8	7	6
Portable Batteries—6 cells—for same	1	1	0
De Zeng's ... Ophthal...scope	10	10	0
The Worth Black Amblyoscope (New Model)	2	10	0
Chambers Inskeep's Gold Medal Ophthalnometer	16	15	0
Geneva ...bined Reti...scope and Ophthalmoscope	16	15	0

PARTICULARS AND PRICES ON APPLICATION—

Sole Importing Agents:

A. E. STALEY & Co.,
19, THAVIES INN, LONDON, E.C.

The Luminous Ophthalmoscope.

All our preparations bear our special label.
BEWARE OF IMITATIONS.

ALYPIN.

A NEW LOCAL ANÆSTHETIC.

Qualified in a remarkable degree to

REPLACE COCAINE IN ALL CASES.

Less toxic and occasioning no mydriasis, and no disturbance of accommodation.

Dose: Corresponds with that of Cocaine.

Can be sterilised and combined with supra-renal preparations.

PROTARGOL.

An organic silver preparation in
EYE DISEASES.
Excellent results obtained in Blennorrhoea
Neonatorum, Conjunctivitis, Dacryocystitis,
etc.
To be applied in 2-20 per cent. solutions.

ASPIRIN.

An excellent substitute for the salicylates,
in rheumatic affections of the eye,
(iritis, cyclitis, glaucoma, &c.),
without the bad after-effects of the latter.
DOSE—15 grains, 3-5 times daily.

For Free Samples and Literature apply to:
THE BAYER CO., Ltd., 19, St. Dunstan's Hill, LONDON. E.C.

Transactions of the Ophthalmological Society of the United Kingdom.

—

FULL PRICE will be given for Volumes I., II.,
III., and VI., if in good condition.

Apply—SIGNA,

OPHTHALMOSCOPE OFFICES,

24, Thayer Street,

LONDON, W.

ADVERTISEMENTS.

iii.

IN THE TREATMENT OF

ANÆMIA, NEURASTHENIA, BRONCHITIS, INFLUENZA, PULMONARY
TUBERCULOSIS, AND WASTING DISEASES OF CHILDHOOD, AND DURING
CONVALESCENCE FROM EXHAUSTING DISEASES,

THE PHYSICIAN OF MANY YEARS' EXPERIENCE

KNOWS THAT, TO OBTAIN IMMEDIATE RESULTS, THERE IS NO REMEDY THAT
POSSESSES THE POWER TO ALTER DISORDERED FUNCTIONS LIKE

Fellows' Syrup of Hypophosphites"

MANY A TEXT-BOOK ON RESPIRATORY DISEASES SPECIFICALLY MENTION
THIS PREPARATION AS BEING OF STERLING WORTH

TRY IT, AND PROVE THESE FACTS.

SPECIAL NOTE.—Fellows' Syrup is never sold in bulk, but is dispensed in bottles
containing 8 oz. and 15 oz.

This preparation may be obtained at all Chemists and Pharmacists throughout
United Kingdom.

TO THE

Eye, Ear. Nose &

Throat Profession:

SEND FOR MY
LAST BULLETIN.

I have in Stock APPROVED
SPECIALITIES in

INSTRUMENT and
APPARATUS . . .

in your line, and shall be pleased
to supply your wants.

Joseph C. Ferguson, Jr., (Optician to Wills Hospital) 8 & 10, Sth. 15th Street,
PHILADELPHIA.

THE UNIQUE VALUE OF

ARGYROL (SILVER VITELLIN)

In ocular therapeutics has been attested to at all recent ophthalmolog
congresses by the most conservative ophthalmic surgeons.

ITS NON-IRRITATING CHARACTER—A SEVERE TEST

Dr. EDGAR S. THOMSON, New York, Surgeon to Manhattan F
and Ear Hospital, stated in a paper read before the Medical Society
the State of New York:

"When a non-irritating germicide is required, Argyrol is certainly ideal.
have recently seen injected a 25 per cent. solution into the anterior chamber of
infected eye with remarkable checking of the process, and without the sligh
irritation to the iris."

Dr. S. LEWIS ZIEGLER, of Philadelphia, Surgeon to Wills' E
Hospital, writes concerning the treatment of corneal ulceration :

Argyrol, in strengths of 10 to 20 per cent., proves beneficial both by
antiseptic action on the ulcer itself, and also by its sedative action on the corn
It possesses the important advantage of causing neither pain nor irritation.'

Dr. D. K. SHUTE, Ophthalmologist to Maternity Hospital, etc., Was
ington, D.C., writes :

"I have recently observed twenty-one cases of ophthalmia neonatorum
which the other means ordinarily employed had little effect on the purulent proce
but in which Argyrol proved efficient. Under the use of 25 per cent. solution
Argyrol, the pus was gotten under absolute control in from forty-eight to seventy-t
hours. It is also the best antiseptic we have for use before cataract operations."

HOW TO USE ARGYROL:

Purulent conjunctivitis (gonorrhœal, neonatorum, etc.), free instillation of 25 per ce
solution every 3 or 4 hours ; catarrhal conjunctivitis, 5 to 20 per cent. one or more times dai
trachoma, 25 per cent. solution rubbed with force into lids once daily ; dacryocystitis, corn
ulcers, etc., 25 per cent. solution.

It is not necessary to remove excess of Argyrol with salt solution

Argyrol is freely soluble in all proportions of water. The solutions keep indefinitely

PRODUCED BY

BARNES & HILLE, 32, Snow Hill, London, E.C

Furnished only in 1-oz. bottles. Price to Physicians, 5/6 per bottle.

THE
OPHTHALMOSCOPE.
A MONTHLY REVIEW OF CURRENT OPHTHALMOLOGY.

VOL. III.—No. 12.] *DECEMBER 1, 1905.* [ONE SHILLING

CONTENTS.

ORIGINAL COMMUNICATIONS.

ON MENINGITIS FOLLOWING EXCISION OF THE EYEBALL.

BY

C. DEVEREUX MARSHALL, F.R.C.S.

ASSISTANT SURGEON ROYAL LONDON OPHTHALMIC HOSPITAL (MOORFIELDS);
OPHTHALMIC SURGEON VICTORIA HOSPITAL FOR CHILDREN, LONDON,
HON. SECRETARY OPHTHALMOLOGICAL SOCIETY OF THE UNITED KINGDOM.

Considering the large number of eyeballs which have been removed for injury and disease, and considering also the close proximity of the brain and meninges, and the fact that the optic nerve is really a prolongation of the brain, and its sheath a prolongation of the meninges, it is perhaps a matter of surprise than otherwise to note how seldom it happens that meningitis follows panophthalmitis. Septic diseases are now so effectually combated, that a surgeon, if not the patient and friends, would consider it little short of a crime were such a disease as erysipelas to follow an operation which was undertaken on uninfected tissues, for one's power of preventing such developments is probably as perfect as it ever will be, and nothing but carelessness on the part of the surgeon or his assistants would be now likely to lead to such a result.

With the eye things are rather different. It is impossible at any time to render the conjunctival sac absolutely aseptic, and if this were accomplished, and the integrity of the eye at the same time retained, there would still be a direct communication with the nose by means of the canaliculus and nasal duct, which would be a grave source of re-infection. In this way the ophthalmic surgeon is at a disadvantage, and is often accused of being careless in the rules he observes and the precautions he practises. Thus, we see most scrupulous attention paid by the general surgeon, not only to purifying his hands, putting on rubber gloves, etc., but even to having sterilised culture-tubes inoculated from his hands, in order to see if any organisms still survive the severe treatment to which they have been subjected. His clothes are also completely covered with a sterilized garment, and with the field of operation surrounded by similar things, it is almost impossible for him to re-infect his hands once they are rendered aseptic.

It is comparatively seldom that such elaborate precautions are taken by the ophthalmic surgeon, and it is indeed difficult to say what good would result if he did. It certainly is well to eliminate all possible sources of infection, and to avoid every appearance of evil ; however, considering the fact that the surgeon's fingers are never used in an intraocular operation, except in the way of holding the handle of an instrument, or when handling needles or sutures, it can make but little difference to the eye whether he has gone to the full length of the extensive sterilization of his hands that are so essential for the success of a general surgical operation, where the hands are, perhaps, in direct contact with the wound. No one has, I think, ever suggested that the eyelids can be thoroughly sterilized, and the ready way in which operation wounds heal up in the lids could scarcely be expedited or rendered more satisfactory if the parts could be rendered surgically clean.

With regard to intraocular operations, it is the custom of some surgeons to have the conjunctival sac examined bacteriologically before they will undertake the removal of, say, a cataract. This is no doubt an excellent precaution. It must impress the patient immensely, and probably very rightly lead him to think that the surgeon considers no detail too small to insure the success of the operation. Still, with all this, it is exceedingly difficult, when looking at a crop of organisms from the conjunctiva, which are practically always present, to say that in this preparation they are all harmless, or in another they are all, or any of them, dangerous, and I have little doubt but that the occasional suppuration of an eyeball will follow the performance of an intraocular operation, no matter how long the surgeon may have had the good fortune to escape such a disaster, and no matter how firmly he may believe in his own methods, as being essential to ensure the prevention of such a disaster.

In this communication I do not wish to confine myself entirely to suppuration after operation, but to discuss the whole subject of panophthalmitis, and the immediate and remote effects of this disease, together with its best and most rational treatment.

It is so well recognised that fatal meningitis may occasionally follow enucleation of an eyeball in a state of suppuration, that it has become almost an axiom with some surgeons that when panophthalmitis is present, the eye should not be removed. The common idea is that under such circumstances the only thing that should be done is to make an incision into the eyeball and let what will come away. Then, a certain period of time is allowed to elapse until the globe becomes a more or less shrivelled mass, when it may, with safety, be removed. Other operators will venture farther, and will not only incise the eye, but will scrape away the suppurating contents. By either of these procedures, the supporters of the method claim that meningitis is most likely to be avoided.

The grounds on which this claim is made are doubtless reasonable enough, for the advocates claim exemption from this dread disease after such treatment, although it is certainly difficult to see what good can accrue to the patient by having a mass of suppurating vitreous and choroid left within his sclerotic. The fact of leaving it open to the air, although it may aid drainage, is not likely to render it less septic. In addition, during the whole time that pus is present, there must be a risk of its soaking backwards and infiltrating the orbit, as, indeed, we know it does, and proof of this is easily seen in the matted and hardened tissues that are present when we excise such an eye. It is absurd to say there is no danger in this, since we may easily get the veins thrombosed with septic clot, and portions may be washed backwards into the circulation, and thus lead not only to septic meningitis, but even to pyæmia, which is always a possibility whenever an abscess is present containing septic pus. In addition to this, there is the lymph-stream to consider, and we all know how readily septic material may be carried by the lymphatics, as is shown by the enlarged and suppurating glands that may follow a septic sore on the hand or foot. It is thus obvious that if meningitis does not occur under these circumstances, it is certainly not because the local conditions are unfavourable ; they are, in fact, most likely to produce it. The advocates of excision of a suppurating eyeball are in a far stronger position theoretically, for they claim that the presence of septic material within the eye is a very real source of danger, and the longer it is left the greater will be the probability of its becoming disseminated. Let us, however, look for a moment at the conditions which exist when such an eye is removed.

If the operation is undertaken as soon as suppuration is well established, there is a chance, in many instances, of removing the globe without allowing any of the inflammatory contents to escape. We are thus able to excise the abscess, walls and all, and the only direct communication with the brain which exists is along the sheath of the optic nerve. If, however, this stage is passed, we may find the orbital fat infiltrated with inflammatory material, and the contents of the eye may escape through a rupture of the globe during operation, or from a wound which has insecurely healed.

Here, undoubtedly, is a source of danger, for we not only stir up the parts that are already inflamed, but we also flood the recently cut tissues with the purulent contents of the eyeball, and it is not difficult to understand that septic organisms have thereby a very easy route opened to them into the meninges. On the other hand, there is never the smallest necessity to run this risk, for no matter how badly the eye is injured, it is always possible to remove the contents, and thoroughly to disinfect the conjunctival sac and the interior of the eye by the application of strong antiseptic solutions, which in this case may be used in as powerful a form as they can be applied to any other part of the body, inasmuch as we have no clear cornea to take into consideration. Immediately this has been done, the sclerotic can be excised, and no risk will be run of infecting the deeper parts. It may be urged, why not be content with eviscerating the globe only ; the sclerotic may then be excised later, if necessary. This might certainly be done, but what possible good could a shrunken sclerotic be to anyone, and if it be thoroughly soaked in septic discharges it may still contribute a fresh dose of poison to the tissues surrounding it, while the risk of removing it at the time can certainly be no greater than making another operation of it at a later date.

If an eyeball be removed with an average amount of skill, as it would be by an experienced operator, there are remarkably few globes that burst while being excised, no matter how badly they may have been injured. I admit that every now and then one comes across an eye that cannot be removed without its contents escaping, although in nine cases out of ten it is caused by a careless or clumsy operator, and need not otherwise happen. Still, if it is likely to occur we had far better make no bones about it, but start by cutting away the cornea and then thoroughly clearing out everything that lies within the sclera.

It may be said, if you consider excision of the eyeball a safe operation, how do you account for the fact that several cases of death have been recorded after the removal of suppurating eyes, while few have occurred when they have been left. The explanation is simple. There are few who consider it safe to leave a putrid mass in such close proximity to the brain, and by far the greater number of such eyes are excised, and I maintain that the patients who die from meningitis after excision do so because the eye was left long enough to produce the disease before it was removed. I have myself known and recorded several cases in which meningitis followed suppuration of the eyeball when the eye was not operated upon at all. Two cases of this nature are mentioned in a paper, published by me, in the *Royal London Ophthalmic Hospital Reports*, vol. XIV, p. 312. The first was a case recorded by Mr. Waren Tay in vol. VII, p. 506, of the same *Reports*, and occurred in a woman, aged 68 years, whose cataractous lens had been removed two years before. Glaucoma then developed, and consequently an iridectomy was done. After the operation the eye suppurated, and the patient died thirteen days later. There was extensive suppurative meningitis ; the ventricles contained purulent fluid ; and there were many hæmorrhages over the brain. In the posterior part of the left orbit was an abscess containing blood-stained pus. It will be noticed that in this case the eye was not removed during life.

In another case, described in detail in the same paper, the patient was aged ten months. One eye suppurated from an unknown cause ; later broncho-pneumonia developed, and the child died. The eye was not removed, but all the same the patient died from purulent meningitis, which was found to extend on to the surfaces of both hemispheres and down to the base. There was no excess of fluid in the ventricles, and no tubercle. The whole of the vitreous was suppurating.

In many of the recorded cases of death from meningitis after excision, the patients have shown all the symptoms of early meningitis before the eye was removed, and the fact that meningitis may be present for a considerable time without any symptoms whatever, is very well known. I gave details of one remarkable case of this kind in the paper previously mentioned. Aural surgeons are very well acquainted with this in those sad cases in which the disease follows suppuration of the middle ear. If we were to admit that removing a suppurating eye was a dangerous proceeding, we should be forced to admit also that opening a mastoid in a similar condition was equally likely to produce the same disease.   It seems to me that one view is as untenable as the other.

A case in which death occurred after enucleation of a suppurating eye has recently been published by Enslin and Kuwahara (*Archiv für Augenheilkunde*, Sept., 1904*), which they state points strongly to the view that suppurating eyes should not be removed.   The patient was a woman, aged 64, whose eye had been chonically inflamed for a year or more after an infective corneal ulcer.   The eye was quite blind and very painful.   It was decided to remove it.   At the operation the conjunctiva was found to be adherent to the eyeball, and no doubt the tissues behind the globe were also infiltrated.   The eye was perforated during the operation, with the result that some of the contents escaped into the orbit.   Symptoms of acute meningitis rapidly followed, and the patient died fifty-eight hours later.   Streptococci were found in the globe, and likewise in the washings from the orbit taken before death.   There was no evidence of acute inflammation of the orbit ; streptococci were present in the nerve sheath ; and chronic interstitial inflammation of the nerve itself was found.   The *post-mortem* condition of the brain we are not told, but I should have but little doubt but that the surfaces of the hemispheres were largely affected, and had probably been so for weeks, although this is, of course, only surmise, but founded on the many similar cases I have seen and heard about ; probably, also, a fresh dose of poison was admitted from the organisms which were let free from the interior of the eyeball.   Here, now, is a typical instance of death occurring from faulty treatment.   Very possibly the surgeons had not the chance of operating before, but whether they had, or had not, the facts obviously point to the conclusion that the patient died because a suppurating eye was left too long. In an abstract of this paper, published in the *Ophthalmic Review* for March, 1905, the reviewer states that this paper "is entirely opposed to the position taken up by Marshall in advocating enucleation."   I am, however, quite content in putting it forward as a case entirely favouring the view I hold.   If this eye had not been removed, the patient would have been worn out with pain, and I should with confidence have expected her to die from meningitis had she been left alone, although I think it more than likely that the clumsy way in which the eye was removed, and the fresh-cut tissues were infected, hastened the process.   Such an eye ought never to have been left so long ; it should have

---

*For abstract see THE OPHTHALMOSCOPE, May, 1905, *p*. 235.—EDITORS.

been excised weeks or months before ; still, had such a case come under my care, I should have excised it whenever I saw it, no matter how long it had been suppurating, and I should not have felt justified in waiting a single hour longer than I was positively obliged. To leave such an eye is opposed to all sound principles of surgery, and reminds one of nothing so much as the antiquated, although popular, notion that an abscess had best be left to burst itself, and that a tooth causing an alveolar abscess should not be removed until the swelling had gone down. For some years past I have never seen a suppurating eye without advising its immediate removal, and of all the hundreds that have come under my notice in this condition, I have never once regretted the opinion I have held.

It has been held, that if such an eye be excised, it is dangerous to irrigate the orbit afterwards, because it may assist the dissemination of the organisms. If the fluid were pumped under pressure into a closed cavity it certainly might do so, but it is irrational to hold that irrigation of a cut and possibly septic surface with an antiseptic solution can in any way aid the development and dissemination of organisms, and this is the thing I always do if there be reason to suppose that the orbital tissues are already infiltrated.

It is never necessary to apply a tight bandage after excision except for the first hour or two. After the bleeding has ceased, which it will invariably have done after this time, a light pad and bandage are all that is necessary, and it is especially advisable to insure free drainage and irrigation after the removal of a suppurating eye. I feel sure that in this way meningitis and death may frequently be avoided.

SOME UNUSUAL FUNDUS CONDITIONS.

BY

ALEXANDER DUANE, M.D.,

NEW YORK CITY, U.S.A.

I. Black Spot at the Macula in Myopia.

The occurrence of a sharply-defined, circular black spot in the macula of myopic eyes has been signalised by various authors, notably by Fuchs, who has given a very clear account of the symptoms, course, and ophthalmoscopic appearances.

The cases are probably not very rare, and the only interest attached to those subjoined is, that in the first I had the rather unusual opportunity of seeing the patient both directly before, and also directly after, the development of the black spot, and was thus able to note the immediate effect produced by it on the vision. The second case was somewhat peculiar, in that the spot, although in other respects typical, was evidently not quite at the macula, and thus did not produce the usual great reduction of central vision.

CASE I.—PROGRESSIVE MYOPIA ; DEVELOPMENT OF BLACK SPOT IN MACULA WITH SUDDEN REDUCTION OF VISION.— Samuel S. H., *ætat* 36, under homatropine :

Right c.—-16.00D. 15/30 +
Left   c.—12.00—3.00 cyl. 20°, 15/30+

From the history of previous examinations, it is evident that myopia has advanced 2 dioptrics in the last three years. Had worn under-correcting glasses for distance, and weaker glasses still for near.

In the fundus of both eyes, numerous, scattered, patchy accumulations of pigment and a terraced temporo-annular conus. In right eye also a spot of choroidal atrophy below the macular region, and a small spot of atrophy to nasal side of disc.

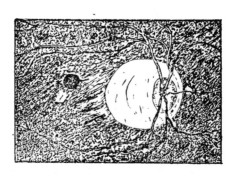

FIG. I.

R. eye in Case I. ; previous examination showed exactly the same except the black spot. No attempt has been made to reproduce vessels precisely, but otherwise representation fairly accurate, except that central spot was blacker than is shown in the drawing.

Two months later patient came in, stating that for one month he had noticed blurring of sight when left eye was shut, but not with both eyes open. R. with his glasses 5/200 (by slightly eccentric fixation, 15/200). Absolute central scotoma, about 3° in diameter. Fundus just as before, except that in macula there is a round spot of blackish pigment, somewhat thinned, and lighter coloured in the centre (*see* FIG. I).

CASE 2.—EXTRA-MACULAR BLACK SPOT WITH MYOPIA ; COMPARATIVELY GOOD CENTRAL VISION.

Amelia R.,*ætat* 31 years.

Right c.—13·00, $\frac{20}{40}$

Left c.—19·00, $\frac{20}{70}$

Sharp, silvery-white, temporal conus, right and left ; spotty scattered pigmentation, but no rarefaction outside of conus. In left eye, horizontal oval black spot, like an ink blot, with palish centre, about $\frac{1}{5}$ the diameter of the disc, lies below and somewhat to the nasal side of the macula.

II. Coloboma of Macula.

CASE 3. — COLOBOMA OF CHOROID AND RETINA SKIRTING MACULA ; PARA-CENTRAL SCOTOMA.

Ernest B., *ætat* 30, accidentally noticed, fifteen years ago, that he could not see well when he shut the right eye, although he could see well with both eyes open.

R. (under homatropine) c. + 0·50 + 0·50 cyl. 110° 15/10. L. 15/40 to 15/100 ; no glass improves, but skiascopy shows + 0·75 cyl. 120°. L., absolute scotoma beginning 2° to the nasal side of fixation point and extending nasally 21°. Central vision

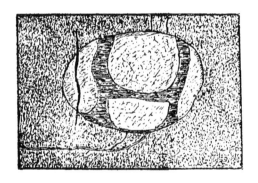

FiG. 2.

somewhat indistinct (relative central scotoma). Outside of scotoma all colors perceived normally and peripheral field for small dot normal.

In left eye, slightly below the macula, undermined oval pit, four to five disc-breadths wide and five to six disc-breadths long, enclosing four mottled white patches of sclera (*See* Fig. 2). These appear to be about 1 mm. below the level of the surrounding fundus. One pigment stripe crosses the innermost patch. Otherwise no pigment patches and no pigment border to coloboma. No retinal vessels traverse the area, although some are cut short right at the margin of the pit. One or two choroidal vessels visible in the latter.   The rest of the fundus, including the disc, normal.   No temporal pallor of disc.

CASE 4.—COLOBOMA OF CHOROID IN MACULAR REGION WITH PARTIAL RETENTION OF RETINA.

Grace D., *ætat* 30 years.   R., 20/20 ; under homatropine, hyperopia 1 D. ; eye normal in all respects.   L., 20/20 ; under homatropine, hyperopia of 0.75 D.   Field (*see* Fig. 3) uniformly contracted down to about 20 degs.

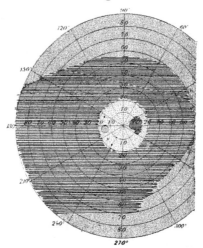

FIG. 3.

Within this area one or two small, scattered scotomata and one large scotoma on nasal side.   Egg-shaped coloboma in macula, 2.5 by 1.0 disc-breadths in size (*see* Fig. 4).   Covering rounded

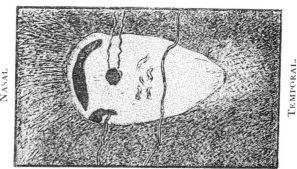

FIG. 4.

nasal end is heavy, coal-black pigment stripe ; at lower border irregular pigment patch (both patches really blacker than represented in drawing).   A large retinal vein (secondary branch of papillary vein) runs to this and is lost upon it.   Another pigment heap in centre of coloboma. Two fine retinal vessels run out to this and are lost under it. Another retinal vessel crosses coloboma at temporal end. On floor of coloboma several worm-like remains of vessels (apparently choroidal). Choroid near temporal end of coloboma attenuated, and near nasal end shows radial striation; otherwise normal, except for pigment heaps above noted. No accumulations of pigment on border of coloboma or elsewhere. Optic nerve normal ; no temporal pallor.

III. Coloboma of Choroid with Filament projecting from it into Vitreous.

CASE 5.—George A. M., *ætat* 27 years, gradually failing vision in right eye. R., 20/200 varying. L., with slight astigmatic correction, 20/20. Right central scotoma about 5 degs. in extent.

In the right eye below the disc is a coloboma of the choroid

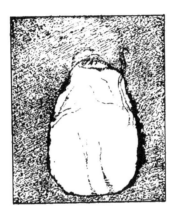

FIG. 5.

of ordinary appearance, with heavily pigmented edges and with some rarefaction of the adjacent choroid. Attached to the nasal border of this by very fine filaments, resembling the byssus of a mussel, is a slender, transparent, elongated, worm-like body which extends out a short distance (seemingly not over 1 mm.) into the vitreous, and then apparently runs parallel to the plane of the retina. Its free end is bent back, sharp, and hook-like. This body lies free in the vitreous, and while usually fixed, sometimes makes slight wavy movements, even when the patient's head is steady. On account of its transparency it is very difficult to see (*see* Fig. 5., in which the distinctness of the filament has been exaggerated purposely, in order to show its situation and attachment).

The poor central vision and central scotoma, as subsequent examinations showed, were due to a central choroiditis which produced a faint striate atrophy in the macula. No changes were observed in the vicinity of the coloboma or its appendage during the seven years that the patient was under observation.

UPON DISSEMINATED SYMPATHETIC CHOROIDITIS.

BY

DR. HENRI COPPEZ,

AGRÉGÉ À L'UNIVERSITÉ DE BRUXELLES.

In addition to the classical forms of sympathetic ophthalmitis, plastic and serous iridocyclitis, there exists a variety which is rarer, but still sufficiently characterized to merit a special description. This variety is disseminated choroiditis of sympathetic origin.

This affection manifests itself by the appearance of little, round spots of yellowish colour in the periphery of the choroid. These are very small, measuring scarcely $\frac{1}{10}$ of the papillary diameter; they are of nearly equal dimensions, but at times some become confluent in such a way as to form a focus of some little size with festooned edges. They are to be found more particularly near the branches of the retinal vessels, which often cross them. Their border is regular— not encircled by pigment.

There is generally little effect on the neighbouring parts. The papilla is slightly hyperæmic; the veins are more or less dilated. The vitreous body remains transparent. The iris does not present anything special; there is sometimes a little Descemetitis. Perikeratitic injection is absent or very slight.

After several months, these deposits disappear, leaving behind no traces, or they become atrophic; they bleach, but without abnormal pigmentation; others persist without modification.

The prognosis is favourable. The greater part of the cases known have recovered. Atropine and mercurial injections are recommended, and, above all, a prolonged sojourn in a darkened room.

The usual forms of sympathetic ophthalmitis are sometimes accompanied by similar lesions. Then, however, there must be a concurrence of favourable circumstances in order to recognise the deposits. The media must be clear enough in such a case to render ophthalmoscopic examination possible, which is, unhappily, not always the case. This disseminated choroiditis, whatever it may be, does not resemble any other form of choroiditis. It is characterized by the smallness and regularity of the spots; their arrangement behind the terminal ramifications of the retinal vessels; and by the absence of pigment. It is somewhat difficult to explain the mode of formation of these foci. S. Osaki (*loco citato*), who has observed a similar case in the Marburg clinic, believes that irritating substances, parts of the iris and of the ciliary body, go backwards, carried along by the lymphatic current. The lymphatic passages surround the vessels. In places they enclose little accumulations of lymphoid cells. These accumulations, under the action of irritating substances, develop exactly like the lymphatic ganglia, and thus become visible under the ophthalmoscope.

The cases of disseminated sympathetic choroiditis hitherto published are few. The following may be briefly cited :--

1. **Eversbusch**. — (*Mittheil. aus der Univ. Augenkl. München*, I, 1882). Young girl, *ætat* 22 years. Enucleation of the sympathising eye. Complete cure in several weeks. The spots disappeared completely.

2. **Dolschenko**.—(*Russische Zeitschrift für Ophthalmologie*, 1884. Ref. *Centralbl. f. prak. Augen.*, 1885, p. 387). Two cases of sympathetic ophthalmia, with some foci of disseminated choroiditis.

3. **Leplat.**—(*Annales de la Société médico-chirurgicale de Liége*, No. 1, 1888). Chorio-retinitis occupying the lower half of the globe, with disappearance of the corresponding visual field. The lesions were not so characteristic as in the other cases.

4. **Schirmer.**—(*Archiv für Ophthalmologie*, xxxviii, 4, page 95, 1892). Man, *ætat* 20 years. Sympathising eye atrophied. Troubles of the vitreous body in the other eye, with an accumulation of atrophic pigment and spots in the choroid.

5. **Hirschberg.**— " *Ueber sympathische Augenentzündung.*" (*Centralbl. f. prak. Augenheilk.*, 1895, p. 80). The author remarks that the same foci can be found in the wounded eye. This case concerns a little girl, *ætat* 6 years. The sympathising eye was not enucleated. The evolution had not stopped at the time of the publication of the article.

6. **Caspar.**—" *Chorioiditis disseminata sympathica.*" (*Klin. Monatsbl. f. Augenheilk.*, 1895, p. 179). Child, *ætat* 9½ years. The largest foci, which, however, do not exceed ⅙ diameter of the disc, enclosed in the centre a little pigmented spot. There was never an edging of pigment. The affection dated from 3½ years of age The acuity of vision was satisfactory. The injured eye had not been enucleated, but was atrophied.

7. **Haab.**—(*Ophth. Gesell. Heidelberg*, 1897, p. 165), Report of four analogous cases. The faithful reproduction of

one of these cases is to be found in Schirmer's " Sympathische Augenerkrankung," Graefe-Saemisch, *Handbuch der Gesamten Augenheilkunde*, 2 Aufl., 23rd part, and in Haab's Atlas of Ophthalmoscopy, 2nd part, Fig. 39).

8. **Osaki.**—(*Arch. f. Augenheilk.*, XLV, p. 126, 1902.) Man, *ætat* 31 years. Cured sympathetic iridocyclitis. Characteristic spots in the choroid.

Personal Observations.

1st Case —Alfred D., *ætat* 17 years, was wounded in the left eye on 15th December, 1904. while handling a kitchen knife. When, on the following day, he came to consult me. I found a very extended wound, 3 c m. long. in a half circle, involving the sclerotic and the cornea. On the level of the limbus, the iris had a very pronounced prolapse. The crystalline lens was opaque ; the tension was reduced to the minimum. There was no perception of light. On 17th December, the herniated parts of the iris were excised ; 17th January, 1905, the patient left the clinic in good health. A little circumcorneal injection, however, persisted.

On the 10th February, I found the left eye atrophied, injected, and painful on pressure. The iris was of a dirty colour ; violent headaches. As regards the right eye, there existed very slight pericorneal injection ; the pupil re-acted normally. With Berger's binocular-glass, however, one could verify several minute grey spots upon the posterior surface of the cornea. The visual acuity was normal. With the ophthalmoscope, one could discover nothing suspicious ; the papilla has its usual appearance.

Enucleation was performed the same day. The patient was put into a darkened room, and subjected to mercurial friction daily. Under the action of the atropine the pupil was dilated to its maximum. From March 2nd. there were added to the treatment sub-conjunctival injections of chloride of sodium, 2%, from day to day. At the same time there was found in the lower part of the choroid, towards the equator, a series of very small spots, measuring scarcely $\frac{1}{10}$ or $\frac{1}{20}$ of the papillary diameter. There were about twenty of these spots, which were sometimes confluent, and formed then a festooned *plaque.* They were situated principally behind the retinal veins. There were no opacities in the vitreous body. The visual acuity was normal. The tension was good.

On the 25th March the papilla has resumed its normal aspect. The atropine has been discontinued for ten days. There was no longer perikeratitic injection or corneal deposits. In May the cure was maintained, half of the choroiditic spots were effaced. The others persisted without any change. There was neither atrophy nor pigmentation.

2nd Case —L. Lucien, farrier, *ætat* 36 years. wounded July 19th, by a fragment of hot iron. On the following day, on the arrival of the patient at the clinic, there could be diagnosed, apart from a slight burn of the eye-lashes. a linear wound, several millimetres in length, occupying the ciliary zone of the sclerotic. Through this wound, which was situated immediately above the cornea, the iris had prolapsed. The perception of light was satisfactory. There were orbital and periocular pains.

After several days the wound cicatrised, and the patient left. He came again on September 9th, in order to undergo an iridectomy, the eye having become the seat of some glaucomatous phenomena. The operation was carried out without incident, and the patient went out on September 24th. He returned on October 10th, the left eye having become very painful. It was markedly injected ; the vision of the other eye was reduced, and the globe was hyperæmic and sensitive to pressure. The eye was enucleated the same day. Despite energetic treatment (atropine, warm compresses, mercurial inunctions, sudorific injections of pilocarpine, darkness) the right eye became the seat of an intense iridocyclitis, with marked pericorneal injection, Descemetitis, and dull papilla. On the 20th October, the fundus of the eye became unilluminable. In the month of November, the mercurial friction was replaced by two injections a week of :—

> Mercury Biniodide, 1 gramme.
> Sodium Iodide, 1 gramme.
> Distilled Water, 50 grammes.
> Dose.—$\frac{1}{2}$ Pravaz syringe.

After several changes, the fundus of the eye cleared up, and in January, 1905, the papilla again became visible.

On July 11th, 1905, I verified the following phenomena :—there was no longer any circumcorneal injection. The pupil was dilated ovally by atropine, which the patient still instils twice a week. There were numerous posterior synechiæ. The Descemetitis had nearly disappeared. The vitreous body contained a fine dust and some translucent membranes. The papilla was normal. In the choroid, towards the periphery, there were little round spots, yellowish in colour, situated behind the retinal veins These spots were absolutely analogous to those described in the first case, but I could discover no more than five or six of them. The acuity of vision was half normal.

CLINICAL, PATHOLOGICAL, AND THERA-PEUTICAL MEMORANDA.

RESTORATION OF SOCKET FOR CARRYING ARTIFICIAL EYE.

BY

ROBERT W. DOYNE, M.A., F.R.C.S.,

READER IN OPHTHALMOLOGY IN THE UNIVERSITY OF OXFORD ; SURGEON TO THE ROYAL EYE HOSPITAL, SOUTHWARK, LONDON.

One hesitates to claim any procedure as new, for often the same idea has occurred to others and has been actually carried out. So far as I know, however, the following operation has not been previously described.

The class of case to which the operation is applicable is that in which the carrying power of the lower lid has been destroyed by wearing an artificial eye that has become rough, or one that has always been a misfit. Under these circumstances, the lid has become everted and flattened, while a mass of cicatricial tissue has often formed upon its surface. The restoration of a lid in this condition is always, I think, a matter of the greatest difficulty. I have known of more than one instance where the mass of cicatricial tissue was excised, in the hope that when the pressure of the adventitious tissue was removed, the scar resulting from excision would draw the lower lid into its proper position. I believe any operation carried out on these lines to be wrong in principle, inasmuch as the mass of newly-formed tissue will disappear of itself to a great extent if no artificial eye be worn for some months. Besides, the operation effects little more than to draw the lower lid somewhat more inwards towards the orbit, without at the same time raising it, so that it can keep an artificial eye in place. It has an additional disadvantage, namely, that the loss of tissue involved in its performance makes subsequent attempts to remedy the defect more difficult.

In the few instances where I have performed the operation to be now described, the results have been uniformly successful, although two of the cases had been treated without benefit by other procedures.

The steps of the operation are briefly as follows :—A large needle, threaded with stout silk, is passed from the conjunctiva of the lid beneath the skin, and made to emerge in the patient's mouth, between the cheek and the gum at a point opposite the angle of the mouth. The needle is withdrawn and threaded with the other end of the silk, and again passed through the conjunctiva, about half an inch away from the first puncture, and made to emerge in the mouth at the same point as the first thread. The two ends of the suture are next tied over a piece of match or rubber tubing, lying between the cheek and the gum, and the match or tubing is twisted two or three times a day, until the silk cuts out. This generally happens in the course of three weeks or so, leaving a band of cicatricial tissue which, by traction at its base, effectually raises the lower lid. The point of entry of the needle should correspond, one to the inner and the other to the outer, side of line of conjunctiva, that is designed for the new sulcus. One must not be too ambitious ; it is better to approach the margin of the lid rather than the depths of the orbit, since in the latter case one might make a deeper sulcus, but the former plan is the more certain.

A good deal of suppuration—the more the better !—occurs in the track of the silk. In one of my cases, an abscess formed on the cheek, which called for incision, but it left a tiny scar only, and in no way prevented a successful result. After the suture has cut out, the stitching of the lids together with a single suture, over a small artificial eye, for two or three weeks, has appeared to me to help to mould the restored portion of the lower lid. A good result, however, can be obtained without having recourse to this second operaton.

OPHTHALMOSCOPIC APPEARANCES OF A CASE OF PERIVASCULITIS OF THE RETINA AND CHOROID:
Gradual Return to the Normal under the Administration of Basham's Mixture.

BY
T. D. MYERS, M.D.
LECTURER ON OPHTHALMOLOGY, U.S NAVAL MEDICAL SCHOOL.

The patient is a young woman, now twenty years of age, who first came under my observation on November 17th, 1897, when a child twelve years of age.

TO ILLUSTRATE DR. MYERS' CASE OF PERIVASCULITIS.

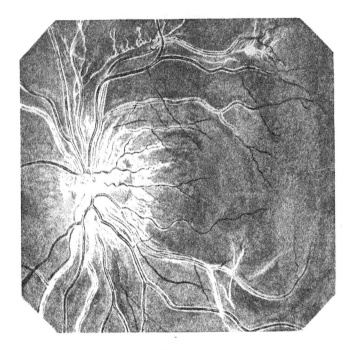

FIG. 1

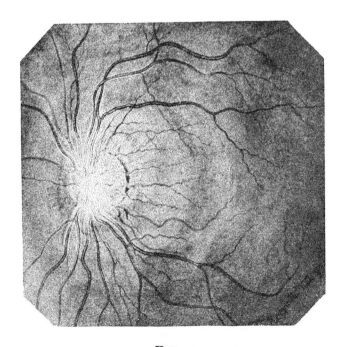

FIG. 2.

She was brought because of some discomfort about her eyes when doing school work. At that time her retinæ were normal in appearance. Her vision was 15/20 with each eye. She had compound hypermetropic astigmatism. Under full atropine cycloplegia, her correction was :—

R.E. + 0·75D. with + 0·75D. Cyl. axis 90° V. = 15/15.
L.E. + 0·50D. with + 0·75D. Cyl. axis 90° V. = 15/15.

She used this correction for near work until October, 1903, when her refraction was again estimated by an cculist in Boston. She states that she never used this last correction, and that she has lost both the glasses and the formula. Between January and March, 1903, she had a swollen gland in the neck, tonsillitis, and an attack of epidemic influenza, and was ill about two months ; she would recover enough to be up and about, and then have a relapse. Her throat was treated in Boston from April till September, when she had the tonsils and the adenoid growths removed by operation. In May, 1904, she had an attack of neuritis of the right arm and forearm, which lasted for six weeks. In December, 1904, she developed a swelling of the right knee joint ; the joint was much swollen but not very painful ; the swelling soon subsided, but was followed by another attack in a less aggravated form, which did not last so long.

The patient again came under my observation on January 14th, 1905. She has developed into a tall, stylish-looking woman, with light hair, blue eyes, and a sallow complexion. She complains that her eyes are not comfortable, and that she has a sensation of strain after using them, especially when sight-seeing or shopping.

Her vision is 15/15 with each eye. She gives a decided family history of gout. She says her right hand shakes after any excitement ; that she is losing weight ; and that she is always tired. Her legs are "boggy" above the ankles ; she has polyuria ; and rises, at least once, every night to pass urine. Heretofore, repeated examinations of her urine have been negative, but in the last examination (May 1st, 1905) minute traces of albumen are reported, but no casts. Heart sounds normal. On examination, her fundi present the remarkable appearance shown in the picture. The perivasculitis is wide-spread throughout both eye-grounds, but is decidedly more marked in the left (see Fig. 1). The lymph-channels of almost every red blood-vessel appear varicose. In many places, partieu-larly in the upper and outer fields of the left eye-ground, fully distended lymph-channels, without visible red-blood vessels, are seen. The distension reaches the peripheral filaments and appears as arborescent terminals. The white striæ are almost solid around the discs, fading off in the surrounding retinæ, like a halo. This condition is well shown in Fig. 1.

The patient was purged with calomel in broken doses, and placed upon a teaspoonful of Basham's mixture,* three times a day.   This treatment was continued for ten days very regularly, but was interrupted at the end of that time by illness and death in her family. She returned to me on March 28th, 1905 ; the change in her eye-grounds was then so striking that I again had them painted by Miss Washington, and the left one is shown in Fig. 2. She resumed the Basham's mixture, and at the moment of writing (May, 1905), the lymph stasis has gradually lessened, but is still quite observable, particularly in the left eye.

It is my impression that the condition has been caused by a gouty exudation into the lymph-channels of the retinal vessels.

AN IMPROVED THERMO-CAUTERY FOR EYE WORK.

BY

SYDNEY STEPHENSON,

LONDON, ENGLAND

IT is needless to speak of the utility of the cautery in eye work, since the fact is widely recognised and fully acted upon by every practical ophthalmologist.   When we turn, however, to the actual instrument employed, there still seems to be room for improvement.   The device of a platinum probe, a squint-hook, or a knitting-needle, heated in a spirit flame, is as unsatisfactory as it is simple.   It may be dismissed without further discussion. The thermo-cautery, in the shape of Paquelin's well-known instrument, is far too cumbersome for the neat performance of the more delicate operations of eye surgery.   Besides, it is not altogether devoid of certain risks connected with the use of a highly explosive liquid like benzine.   These drawbacks have, doubtless, led to the more or less general employment of the galvano-cautery, an admirable appliance, although one not alto-gether devoid of inconveniences.   The current must be supplied from batteries, accumulators, or from the street main.   Batteries and accumulators are cumbersome things to carry about, and never seem to be in working order just when they are most urgently needed.   The employment of the street current implies in the first place that it is laid on ; and, secondly, demands the use of a special convertor costing several pounds.   Lastly, the action of the glowing wire is apt to be hampered by the moist tissues of the eye short-circuiting the current (Haab).

---

* Basham's mixture is a preparation of iron much employed in the United States. It contains tincture of the chloride of iron. 2 parts ; dilute acetic acid, 3 parts ; spirit of Mindererus, 20 parts ; elixir of orange, 10 parts ; syrup, 15 parts ; and water, 50 parts. Dose.—1 to 8 drachms.—EDITORS.

Some little time ago Mr. W. H. Beach brought under the notice of the profession (*Lancet*, December 17th, 1904) a thermo-cautery of simple and ingenious character. The idea, which originated with Paquelin, of keeping a platinum chamber glow-ing by means of hydro-carbon, was retained, but Mr. Beach dis-pensed with the bottle containing the explosive liquid, and in

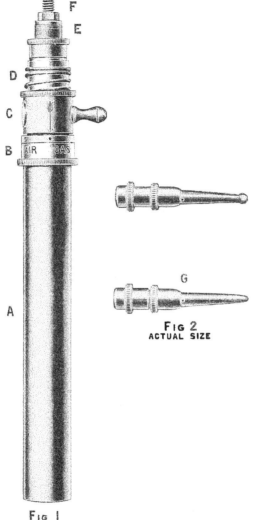

Fig 1
ACTUAL SIZE

Fig 2
ACTUAL SIZE

order to minimise deposit of soot, contrived to aerate the gaseous mixture of hydro-carbon and air. By a simple arrangement he succeeded in regulating with much nicety the proportion of gas and air, thus ensuring a rapid rise in temperature (to 2,000° F. m thirty seconds) in the working point of the new cautery. Other improvements followed, such as a wire gauze screen to prevent the gaseous admixture from exploding or "firing back," and an insulating block, to oppose the maximum degree of resistance to the passage of heat to the stem or handle of the instrument.

A few words of more minute description will render the intimate construction of the thermo-cautery intelligible to readers. The cautery (fig. 2) is made up of the following parts.— The hollow handle (A), which acts as a combined reservoir and vaporizer, is lined with cotton wick, which is saturated with hydro-carbon (petrol) before using the instrument. The trunk (B) comprises an aerator, a refrigerator, a stop-cock, and a collar (C), kept in place by a spring (D). The collar carries an index and an air-tube, the latter forming an attachment for a rubber bellows and tube (not shown in the drawing). A heat-resisting block (E) contains a gauze septum, and a standard (F), to which the working points are secured. The points shown in Fig. 2 are of platinum, hollow, and perforated near the base by a tiny hole (G), through which the products of combustion are blown obliquely backwards.

To work the instrument, the vaporizer (A) is unscrewed, and sufficient petrol is poured into the handle to supersaturate the wick lining, and the excess liquid is returned to the bottle. Having screwed the vaporizer firmly to the trunk (B), the bellows-tube is connected with the nipple. The index, marked by an arrow on the collar (C), is set directly pointing to the tested spot, indicated by a dot engraved upon the trunk (B), the working point is then screwed to the connecting standard (F), and plunged into the spirit-flame for about thirty seconds. As soon as the platinum point has become slightly red, the bellows are squeezed, and the point should glow.

Realising the possibilities in ophthalmic work of this instrument, I suggested to Mr. Beach that a small model should be made for use in eye work. Accordingly he has constructed an instrument (shown above), the length of which is 5 inches, the diameter ½ inch, and the weight 1¼ oz. It is provided with a couple of working platinum ends, one of which is more or less pointed, and the other slightly bulbous (*see* fig. 2). I have found the modified cautery a most efficient instrument, capable of doing whatever the galvano-cautery can effect. A few minutes' experience will allow anybody to use the instrument well. The sole difficulty lies in the exact adjustment of the index, the least variation, even 1/75th of an inch, of which from its proper position over the tested spot would make the platinum point dull in working. Hence, it is advisable, after having once adjusted the instrument precisely, to leave the index arrow in place.

The cautery is packed in a neat wooden case (7in. × 3¾in. × 2in.), which contains, in addition to the cautery itself, a spirit lamp, and a small metallic container for the petrol. The complete outfit can be obtained from Mr. W. H. Beach, Bridgnorth, Salop, England, at a cost of £3 15s. 0d.

NOVELTIES.

A LENS-CENTRING INSTRUMENT.

The correct centring of a spectacle lens is a matter of considerable importance. Faulty centring is not infrequently the cause of discomfort to the spectacle wearer, and it is a fault not always easily detected, especially in the case of oblique, cylindrical, or bifocal lenses.

Messrs. C. W. Dixey & Son, of 3, New Bond Street, and 2c, Welbeck Street, have devised a little instrument which answers admirably the purpose of testing the centring of a spectacle lens. Three points, a perforated disc, a spot on a glass stage, and a cross bar, are set in alignment; an interposed lens disturbs the alignment, which is only restored when the lens is so adjusted that the line of alignment passes through the optical centre. This point is conveniently marked with a glass pencil.

The instrument also contains a scale of angles with a movable cross-bar, so that it may be used to test the setting of cylinder axes.

CURRENT LITERATURE.

NOTE.—Communications of which the titles only are given either contain nothing new or else do not lend themselves to abstract.

1. MALFORMATIONS.

(1) Greeff.—On anophthalmos and other eye deformities and their etiology. (Ueber Anophthalmos mit anderen Missbildungen am Auge und deren Ætiologie.) *Archiv für Augenheilkunde*, 1904, p. 1.

(2) Matys, V.—A malformation of the eye, caused by an amniotic band, in a human foetus of four months. (Eine Missbildung des Auges, bedingt durch ein amniotisches Band, bei einem menschlichen Embryo aus dem vierten Monat.) *Zeitschrift für Augenheilkunde*, Februar, 1905.

(3) Cosmettatos, G. F.—The eye in anencephaly. (De l'œil des anencéphales.) *Archives d'ophtalmologie*, juin, 1905.

(4) **Ovio.**—A case of bilateral anophthalmos. (Caso di anoftalmo bilaterale.) *La Clinica Oculistica*, October, 1905.

(5) **Paramore, R. H.**—A case of anencephalic monster. *Lancet*, October 14th, 1905.

(1) **Greeff** describes a case of anophthalmos, with various other congenital defects, in a female child one and a half years old. There was complete absence of the right globe. The lids were well developed, but the upper punctum was absent, and the eyelashes were practically absent from the lower lid. There was a fairly well-developed conjunctival cavity, but no trace of a globe. Two obliquely-placed bands were found at the outer angle of the eye. The right cheek was more prominent than the left, and there was a large defect in the development of the zygomatic arch, which, however, only slightly affected the orbital margin. On the right side there was slight macrostoma. On the left side of the mouth there was a partial hare lip, and a slight depression on the skin above it leading up a short distance towards the inner angle of the left eye. Both eyelids on this side showed colobomata. The upper eyelid had no punctum. It was present on the lower eyelid, but there was no communication with the nose, and probably no development of a lacrymal duct on that side. The left eye itself was normal. The palate was narrow and high and deeply cleft, and on the right side a bony prominence could be felt which corresponded to the deep depression in the zygomatic arch mentioned above. Greeff, in a very interesting paper, accounts for the development of these various defects by the pressure of amniotic bands in the early stages of fœtal life. He gives two good figures of fœtuses in support of this view. LESLIE PATON.

(2) **Matys** describes in detail the microscopic examination of this interesting malformation, in which it appears that an amniotic band became adherent to the first visceral cleft, and by tension caused an enlargement of the conjunctival sac, and by pressure caused the lids to unite with the sclera and cornea, and at the same time to dislocate forwards the whole eyeball. A. LEVY.

(3) An anencephalous monster, which survived birth nearly five hours, manifested bilateral exophthalmos, and dull and insensitive corneæ. At the autopsy, all internal organs were sound, but the brain was represented by a thin-walled cyst, containing serous fluid. No traces could be found of the chiasma or the intracranial part of the optic nerve. Imperfect medulla present ; spinal cord very small. The eyeballs measured 10mm. by 17mm. by 14mm. The optic nerve, much attenuated, was 18mm. in length, and ended in a fibrous tract at the sella

turcica, without uniting with the opposite nerve to form a chiasma. Microscopical examination of the eye showed, among other things, signs of corneal ulceration, atrophy of iris and ciliary processes, thickened and vascular sclera and choroid, and folded retina, of which the ganglion cells presented an arrest of development, while the layer of nerve-fibres was absent. The hyaloid artery was large and gorged with blood. The optic nerve, composed of vascular connective tissue, contained no nerve-fibres. The vitreous body was made up of slender fibrillæ, anastomosing and forming meshes, filled with a finely granular material. S. S.

(4) **Ovio's** case was an infant who died a few days after birth. The eyelids and palpebral fissure were well formed, though small, but no trace of an eye could be seen. The parts were examined *post mortem*, and complete absence of the eye, optic nerves, chiasma, tracts, and external geniculate bodies were observed. These cases of true anophthalmos are rare ; the arrest of development takes place early during the first few days of fœtal life. The optic vesicles fail to appear, and the other defects are secondary to this. HAROLD GRIMSDALE.

(5) A male fœtus, although otherwise well developed, was born with a peculiar condition of the head. **Paramore** found a normal base, but the rest of the skull was absent, being replaced by two or three black, bulbous, non-pulsating tumours, of semi-solid consistence. These tumours were attached to the base of the skull, where the sella turcica could be recognised with the finger as lying between them. The eyeballs were very prominent owing to the fact that the orbital plates and external angular processes of the frontal bone had not grown forward to cover in the eye, a lack of development due, in its turn, to absence of the frontal lobes of the brain. The mother, 20 years of age, was herself rather a stupid person.

II. AMAUROTIC FAMILY IDIOCY.

(1) Eliasberg, M.—A case of Tay's amaurotic family idiocy. (Ein Fall von Tay-Sachsscher amaurotischer familiärer Idiotie.) *Zeitschrift für Augenheilkunde*, Juni, 1905.

(2) Poynton, F. J. and Parsons, J. Herbert.—Amaurotic family idiocy. *Trans. Ophthalmological Society*, Vol. XXV, 1905.

(1) **Eliasberg** recounts a case of this interesting and rare disease occurring in a family in which at least two other

children (out of seven) suffered from a similar affection. This case is remarkable in its absolutely typical appearances and course.   A. Levy.

(2) **Poynton** and **Parsons** report briefly a typical case of amaurotic idiocy in a Jewish child, aged 13 months.

III. THE SURGICAL TREATMENT OF ASTIGMATISM AND MYOPIA.

(1) Deschamps, D.—Modification of the corneal curvatures under the influence of sub-conjunctival injections; their action on astigmatism. (Modification des courbures de la cornée sous l'influence des injections sous-conjonctivales; leur action sur l'astigmatisme.) *La Clinique Ophtalmologique*, 25 mai, 1905.

(2) Maddox, E. E.—A new operation for moderate short-sight. *British Medical Journal*, October 21st, 1905.

(1) **Deschamps** has satisfied himself that the soldering-down effect of repeated sub-conjunctival injections, so that a dragging action is produced upon the cornea at the site of the injections, results in distinct alteration of the corneal curvature. In the case which first drew the writer's attention to the facts a patient with bilateral H. of 0·50D. came to have H. 2·0D. in the eye which had been treated with injections. Following up this lead, Deschamps proceeded to experiment upon astigmatics with the view of causing flattening of the over-curved meridian. Four cases have been treated in this way with encouraging results. After 18 months two of the cases show a change of refraction of 2D. Full details are not given. Indeed, the author expressly states that he publishes his present observations only in order to draw attention to the matter.   Ernest Thomson.

(2) **Maddox**, in a case of moderate myopia, disqualifying for Woolwich, devised certain operations for the purpose of flattening first one meridian of the cornea and then another at right angles to the first. The following is the method he adopted: he dissected up a flap of conjunctiva in the traverse meridian of the eye, and passed a keratome between the conjunctiva and the sclera into the anterior chamber of the eye. The incision was enlarged above and below with a probe-pointed knife, in order to extend it as much as possible. The second operation, a much simpler affair, was performed 46 days after the first. A large incision was simply made at the lower margin of the cornea with an ordinary cataract knife.

IV. DISLOCATION OF THE LACRYMAL GLAND.

Scrini.—On mobile orbital lacrymal glands. (Des glandes lacrymales orbitaires mobiles.) *Archives d'ophtalmologie*, octobre, 1905.

To the six existing cases of non-traumatic dislocation of the orbital lacrymal gland, Scrini adds a seventh,* the main facts of which follow :—

A man, 44 years of age, developed suddenly and without other symptoms a localised swelling in each upper lid. He had suffered from gonorrhœa six months previously, and two months before the affection of the eyelids was noticed, had fallen from a height of four mètres upon his buttocks. Upon examination, the outer third of the orbito-palpebral groove of each upper lid was effaced by a fold of skin running obliquely from above downwards and from within outwards. The skin presented normal characters. On palpation, the pouch was found to contain a hard, nodular, mobile body, of about the size of a small almond. It was freely movable from side to side, could be reduced temporarily, and was connected with the orbit by a pedicle. No pain or lacrymation. When seen a year after the first examination, the displaced glands had disappeared.

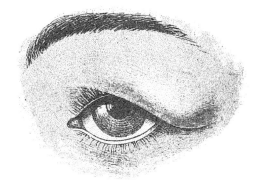

Taking the above case as his text, Scrini discusses many points connected with this singular and rare condition of the lacrymal gland. It may be met with at any age, is more frequent in men than in women, and is generally unilateral. The appearances of the condition are excellently shown in the accompanying illustration, borrowed from a paper by Golovine (*Archives d'ophtalmologie*, 1896, p. 104). The condition is generally discovered by chance. As etiological factors, cough, epilepsy, and violent emotions have been mentioned. Anatomical peculiarities also, may play a part in the production of the luxation, as may augmentation in the volume and weight of the gland. In Scrini's case it is probable that actual dislocation was preceded by chronic inflammation of gonorrhœal origin. S. S.

---

*Scrini, furthermore, gives brief particulars of an eighth case. under the care of Dr. Joseph, where a man of 40 years suffered from bilateral dislocation of the lacrymal glands.

V. ELECTRICITY AND CATARACT.

Desbrières and Bargy.—A case of cataract due to
a discharge of industrial electricity. (Un cas de cataracte
due à une décharge électrique industrielle.) *Annales
d'oculistique*, T. CXXXIII, p. 118, février, 1905.

Desbrières and Bargy record the case of a man who received
a shock from an alternating electric current of 20,000 volts and
30 periods. He was unconscious for half an hour, had severe
burns on the right side of his body, especially the arm and face,
and for the first few days after the accident could not see anything at all with the right eye, owing either to actual loss of
sight or to œdema of the lids, which was so intense as to prevent
an examination of the eyes. A fortnight after the accident,
when the œdema had subsided, the vision of the right eye was
8/10, but objects looked as if seen through a mist; the fundus
was normal; but there were numerous punctiform and linear
opacities in the lens, spread all over its surface, but thickest at
the equator. Eighteen months later, the condition of the eye
was unaltered. The possible explanation of the condition as
due to chemical alteration, destructive action of the current,
circulatory disturbances in the anterior segment of the eye,
or traumatic influence of the current, the prognosis, and the
treatment are discussed.   R. J. COULTER.

VI. SPASMUS NUTANS.

(1) Buchanan, Mary.—Two cases of spasmus nutans.
Annals of Ophthalmology, July, 1905.

(2) Schapringer, A.—On the pathogeny of spasmus nutans.
(Zur pathogenese des Spasmus nutans.) *Centralblatt
für prak. Augenheilkunde*, August, 1905.

(1) Mary Buchanan reports two cases of spasmus nutans and
nystagmus in infants, aged 6 and 7 months respectively, each of
whom had 4 D. of myopia. She assigns this curious affection
to efforts made by the infant to obtain binocular vision, rendered
more difficult than usual by some factor or factors that would
probably be identified, she thinks, if every case was examined at
the outset by an ophthalmologist.

(2) Schapringer discusses the origin of the spasmodic movements of the head accompanied by uni- or bilateral nystagmus
in infants. He agrees with Raudnitz in thinking that the main
cause is keeping children in comparatively dark rooms in which

there are one or more spots of bright light. The infants naturally fix this spot, even if they have to get into uncomfortable attitudes to do so. Raudnitz is of opinion that the fatigue thus brought about is the primary cause of the head movements and, later, of the oscillatory movements of the eye or eyes (binocular vision not being established in infants). Schapringer, on the other hand, is of opinion that fatigue has nothing to do with it, but bases his theory upon the well-known physiological fact of the exhaustion of the retina. Fixation of a bright point rapidly exhausts the corresponding part of the retina, and if the stationary object is still to be seen in all its brightness, it must be fixed by different parts of the retina very frequently, and thus nystagmus is brought about, and, later, spasmodic movements of the head. The condition practically always disappears if the child be kept permanently in well-lit rooms.   A. LEVY.

VII. DISEASES AND MALFORMATIONS OF THE CORNEA.

(1) Stasinski.—A case of neuroparalytic keratitis caused by a periostitis of the upper jaw, with fatal termination. (Ein Fall von Keratitis europaralytica auf Grund einer Periostitis des Oberkiefers mit tödlichen Ausgang.) *Zeitsch. für Augenh.*, Mai, 1904.

(2) Oeller.—Upon acquired pigmentary spots of the posterior wall of the cornea. (Ueber erworbene Pigmentflecke der hinteren Hornhautwand.) *Arch. f. Augenheilk.*, 1903 p. 293.

(3) Zur Nedden.—A case of congenital melanosis corneæ in conjunction with a pigmented reticulation in the anterior chamber, and on the iris. (Ein Fall von angeborener Melanosis Corneæ in Verbindung mit einem Pigmentnetz in der vorderen Kammer und auf der Iris.) *Klin. Montsbl. f. Augenheilk.*, 1903, II, p. 342.

(4) Donaldson, E.—Alveolar sarcoma of the cornea. *Trans. Ophthalmological Society*, Vol. XXIII, 1903.

(5) Ziegler, S. Lewis.—Corneal ulceration due to nasal infection. *American Medicine*, 9th April, 1904.

(6) Velhagen.—On primary striped disturbance of the cornea. (Ueber die primaere bandformige Hornhauttrübung.) *Klin. Monats. f. Augenheilkunde*, 1904, p. 428.

(7) Dor, Louis.—Bilateral keratoconus in the ·course of Basedow's disease, treated on the one side by the actual cautery, disappearing on the other side after treatment with thymus gland directed towards the cure of the Basedow's disease. (Kératocône bilatéral au cours d'une maladie de Basedow, traite d'un côté par la cautérisation ignée et ayant disparu de l'autre côté, par le traitement institué contre la maladie de Basedow, l'opothérapie thymique.) *Revue générale d'ophtalmologique,* juin, 1904.

(8) Jacqueau, A.—Sclerosis of the corneæ in a young subject. (Sclérose des cornées chez un jeune sujet.) *Bull. et Mém. de la Soc. française d'Ophtal.,* 1904, p. 264, and *La Clinique Ophtal.,* 25 juillet, 1904.

(9) Burnett, Swan M.—Appearances simulating optic neuritis due to unsuspected irregular corneal astigmia. *American Journ. of Ophthalmogy,* August, 1904.

(10) Richter, P. V.—A case of hæmorrhagic infiltration of the cornea. (Kasuistischer Beitrag zur Frage der Hornhautdurchblutung.) *Die Ophthalmologische Klinik,* 20 August, 1904.

(11) Lamb, Robert S.—Interstitial keratitis. *Journ. of Eye, Ear, and Throat Diseases,* Sept.-Oct., 1904.

(12) Doyne, Robert W.—A case of ill-developed corneæ. *Trans. Ophthal. Society,* Vol. XXIV (1904), p. 40.

(13) Collins, E. Treacher.—An unusual superficial circumferential opacity of the cornea, symmetrical in the two eyes. *Trans. Ophthl. Society,* Vol. XXIV (1904), p. 45.

(14) Rochat, G. F.—Diplo-bacilli in ulcus serpens. (Diplobacillen bij ulcus serpens.) *Ned. Tijdschrift v. Geneeskunde,* 1904, II, p. 718.

(15) Jocqs, R.—Punctate keratitis. (La kératite ponctuée. *La Clinique ophtalmologique,* 10 décembre, 1904.

(16) Lans, J. L.—Bilateral central fistula of the cornea. (Dubbelzijdige centrale fistel der Cornea.) *Ned. Tijdschrift voor Geneeskunde,* 1904, No. 12.

(17) Cosmettatos.—Papilloma of the bulbar conjunctiva invading the cornea. (Papillome de la conjonctive bulbaire ayant envahi la cornée.) *Ann. d'oculistique,* T. CXXXIII, p. 38, janvier, 1905.

(18) Spicer, W. T. Holmes.—Keratitis profunda. *Ophthalmic Review,* January, 1905.

(19) Wickerkiewicz.—Some considerations upon primary keratoconus. (Quelques considérations sur le kérato-cone primaire.) *Archives d'ophtalmologie,** février, 1905.

(20) Hirschberg, J., and Ginsberg, S.—A rare case of corneal tumour. (Ein seltener Fall von Hornhautgeschwulst.) *Centralbl. für prak. Augenheilkunde*, Februar, 1905.

(21) Vinsonneau, C.—Syphilitic gummata of the cornea. (Gommes syphilitiques de la cornée.) *Archives d'ophtalmologie*, février, 1905.

(22) Jocqs, R.—On keratitis punctata. *Die Ophthalmologische Klinik*, 20 Februar, 1905.

(23) Lauber, Hans.—Upon peripheral ectasia of the cornea. (Ueber periphere Hornhautektasie.) *Klin. Monatsbl. f. Augenheilkunde*, März, 1905.

(24) Paul, L.—On ulceration of the cornea due to diplobacilli. (Ueber Hornhautulcerationen durch Diplobazillen.) *Klinische Monatsblätter für Augenheilkunde*, 1905, XLIII.

(25) Dimmer, F.—A curious persistent change in the cornea after a parenchymatous keratitis. (Eine besondere Art persistierender Hornhautveränderung (Falten-bildung) nach Keratitis parenchymatosa.) *Zeitschrift für Augenheilkunde*, Band. XIII., Ergänzungsheft, 1905.

(26) Dimmer, F.—A form of corneal inflammation resembling keratitis nummularis. (Ueber eine der Keratitis num-mularis nahestehende Hornhautentzündung.) *Zeitschrift für Augenheilkunde*, Band XIII, Ergänzungsheft, 1905.

(27) Wehrli, E.—Nodular opacities of the cornea (Grœnouw) as a primary, isolated, chronic tuberculosis of the anterior layers of the cornea.—(Lupus corneæ, die knötchen-förmige Hornhauttrübung eine primäre, isolierte, chron-ische, tuberkulöse Erkrankung der vorderen Schichten der Cornea.) *Zeitschrift für Augenheilkunde*, April, Mai, und Juni, 1905.

(28) Consiglio, Antonio.—Long interval between parenchy-matous keratitis of the right and left eye. (Langes Intervall zwischen der Keratitis parenchymatosa des rechten und linken Auges.) *Beiträge z. Augenheilkunde*, Mai, 1905.

(29) Campbell, Kenneth.—Acute interstitial keratitis brought on by an injury. *Medical Press and Circular*,17th May,1905.

(30) Posey, W. Campbell.—Keratitis disciformis, with the report of a case. *Ophthalmic Review*, May, 1905.

(31) Terson, A.—Gummata of the cornea. (Les gommes de la cornée.) *Archives d'ophtalmologie*, mai, 1905.

*Wicherkiewicz.—Remarks on primary keratoconus. (Einiges ueber den primären Hornhautkegel.) *Zeitschrift für Augenheilkunde*, February, 1905

(1) **Stasinski** reports the case of a man, aged 45 years, who came to him complaining of some pain and watering of the left eye, with impaired near vision. The trouble had begun about ten days previously, simultaneously with a severe toothache. The left eye, V. $= \frac{5}{75}$, showed slight episcleral injection, anterior chamber somewhat shallow, pupillary reaction sluggish, media clear, tension somewhat raised. The skin supplied by the first and second branches of the trifacial nerve was tender. In the mouth there were a few carious roots, and considerable swelling of the gums on the left side. The diagnosis (subsequently confirmed by Professors Wernicke and Uhthoff, in Breslau) was that of a peripheral ascending inflammation of the fifth nerve, following periostitis of the upper jaw. The patient refused to remain in the hospital, and came up once in ten days. At his next visit a typical ulcus serpens with hypopyon had formed, and a peculiar thickening of the episcleral tissue was found to surround the cornea. This may be looked upon as analogous to the thickenings of the skin found in trifacial affections. At each subsequent visit, patient was found to be worse, and, finally, in about two months from the outset, the author was informed of his death. The diagnosis must have been the correct one, the inflammation travelling up the nerve trunk and finally attacking the base of the brain. The primary increase of tension has been frequently noticed in trifacial affections ; interesting also is the ring-like thickening of the episcleral tissue.   A. LEVY.

(2) **Oeller** has thrice seen pigment spots develop on the membrane of Descemet after intra-ocular operations, and he regards them as pigmented epithelium of the iris, detached by the operation, and adherent to the posterior surface of the cornea.

(3) A patient, of 57 years, complained that for two years his sight had been diminishing in clearness. Examination showed the presence of iridodonesis, cataracta corticalis, and in the anterior chamber a black cobweb-like foreign body, which was connected with numerous little lumps of pigment in the posterior part of the corneal layers. **Zur Nedden** explains the case by supposing a disturbance during embryonic life in the severance of connection between iris and córnea. A. BIRCH-HIRSCHFELD.

(4) **Donaldson** removed an alveolar sarcoma of the cornea in the year 1895 (see *Trans. Ophth. Society*, Vol. XV, p. 90). There was a slight recurrence of the growth four months later, but since then the eye appears to have remained free from the disease.

(5) **Ziegler** considers that fully ninety per cent. of corneal lesions take their origin directly from pre-existent pathologic processes and secretions in the intranasal tissues. He regards the vestibular air spaces as the main receptacles and breeding grounds for the inspired organisms, and, in particular, the maxillary sinus, the special importance and influence of which he discusses in detail. Disease, he says, may be transmitted from the eye to the nose by the nasal duct, by blood and lymph streams, and by reflex action. The first of these paths of disturbance is discussed. Treatment is considered in detail. FRANK W. MARLOW.

(6) **Velhagen** observed in two brothers a central band of discolouration in the cornea of both eyes. Microscopical inspection showed in Bowman's membrane granules deeply coloured with hæmatoxylin or carmine. The granules consisted of chalk, apparently in conjunction with some organic substance. Velhagen considers Leber's explanation to be the correct one, namely, that the chalky deposit was left in the cornea by evaporation of the nutrient fluid, which was abnormally charged with calcareous salts. A. BIRCH-HIRSCHFELD.

(7) A female patient, 24 years old, consulted **Dor** on account of failing vision accompanying Basedow's disease, for which latter she had been treated by various drugs. Dor found that, apart from the usual eye signs of the disease, she also had keratoconus on both sides, that on the left side complicated by a leucoma at its summit. R. V. $\frac{1}{5}$; L. $\frac{1}{20}$. The left conus was treated by the actual cautery, and then, with a view to the cure of the general disease, the patient was ordered to take every day 100 grammes of raw calf sweetbread mixed with sugar and flour. This treatment was successful to a most unexpected degree, for not only did the symptoms of the general disease abate, but the keratoconus on both sides, operated and non-operated, entirely disappeared so that R. V. $= 1$, and L. $= \frac{1}{2}$ (on account of the leucoma). The writer leaves the cause of this remarkable cure open for discussion. ERNEST THOMSON.

(8) A tuberculous girl, 20 years of age, had been subject for sixteen years to slight and transitory attacks of ocular inflammation. Upon examination, **Jacqueau** found a peculiar symmetrical appearance of the corneæ, which presented opaque white circles, having a mother-of-pearl-like sheen, and tending towards a concentric arrangement. The epithelium was intact. Conjunctiva normal. R.V.$=\frac{2}{3}$: L.V.$=\frac{5}{6}$. Local treatment altogether or almost useless. The inflammatory symptoms (never well-marked) disappeared speedily when the patient resided at villages 600 to

800 metres above sea-level. The curious corneal changes—characterised as "sclerosis" by the author—remained without appreciable change during the four years the girl was under Jacqueau's observation.   S. S.

(9) An ophthalmic surgeon had treated a young lady for optic neuritis of one eye, but without tangible result. When the patient was seen by **Burnett**, the sight of the affected eye was 5/15, and there was marked blurring of the retinal vessels · near the upper and. inner edge of the disc. By ordinary methods of examination, no opacity could be detected in either lens or cornea. An investigation by the ophthalmometer, however, at once revealed the character of the trouble. Systematic measurement of the corneal curvature showed that the latter became suddenly more flattened to the nasal side of the centre. In fact, it dropped from 27 at the visual axis to 24 within the first 5, to 21 at 10, to 19 at 20, and to 16 at 20, a total of 11 D. No glass was of service, but with a stenopaic hole, vision rose at once to 5/6.

(10) A baby suffering from general cyanosis (due to congenital heart disease) and from ophthalmia neonatorum, was seen by **Richter** four days after birth. The left cornea then presented the aspect of hæmorrhagic infiltration. The bronze-colour changed from the eighth day into a yellowish-green. The author hints at the possibility of an intra-uterine injury or a connection with the general cyanosis.   C. MARKUS.

(12) **Doyne's** patient, a child of 4 years, showed remarkably flat corneæ, with a faint greyish arcus above and below, extending into the cornea for 2 mm. or 2·5 mm. There was a considerable amount of hypermetropia, with a little astigmatism. No evidence whatever of inherited syphilis.

(13) **Collins's** case occurred in a healthy-looking man, 21 years of age, who showed no signs of hereditary syphilis, either in his physiognomy or teeth. He had been subject for many years to transient attacks of inflammation of the eyes. On ex-amination, Collins found a superficial, greyish, mottled opacity involving the circumference of each cornea, leaving only an oval area of the cornea, a little below the centre, clear and unaffected. No blood vessels were to be recognised in the cornea. The sight was almost normal.

(14) In some cases of serpent ulcer of the cornea with hypopyon, bacilli were observed closely resembling Morax-Axenfeld's diplo-bacilli, but differing from these in their behaviour on culture-media. Thus, they grew abundantly on common agar and gelatine, liquefying the latter, in this respect resembling the "bacillus liquefaciens" found by Petit and

Axenfeld in corneal ulcers. Blood serum was liquefied little or not at all, whereas it ought to be by a true Petit bacillus. Rochat thinks his bacteria a variety of the bacillus liquefaciens. The ulcers in which they were found were remarkably free from pain.   G. F. ROCHAT.

(15) The principal object of this article by **Jocqs** seems to be to show that all forms of so-called punctate keratitis are not dependent upon disease of the uveal tract, but that certain of them are unassociated with any iritis. In these the spots are round, large, and situated in the corneal substance, even towards its anterior surface. The progress may be rapid under local treatment, and the prognosis is favourable.

ERNEST THOMSON.

(16) At the winter meeting of the Dutch Ophthalmological Society **Lans** demonstrated a lady, 44 years old, presenting a corneal cicatrix and anterior synechia on both eyes, as the result of an eye disease contracted, according to the patient herself, after vaccination with human lymph when $2\frac{1}{2}$ years old. She came to consult Lans for a feeling as of a foreign body in her right eye, and on examination, a small prominent vesicle was observed in the centre of the corneal cicatrix; the tension was a little higher than normal. After puncturing this vesicle with a cataract knife, there escaped a small quantity of clear fluid, although the anterior chamber did not become very shallow. After tight bandaging, the eye became normal again in a few days, but a small drop of clear fluid could be seen filtering through the fistula every now and then. In the left cornea a similar vesicle was occasionally observed, disappearing after massage and bandaging. The case was one of bilateral fistula. So long as the fistulæ allowed a small quantity of fluid to escape, the eyes caused no discomfort, but every time the tiny opening was closed, the tension rose and a vesicle formed. After puncturing the latter, the normal condition was restored.

The patient, as mentioned above, attributed her disease to inflammation of the eyes following vaccination with human lymph. If there really exists a connexion, what can the original disease have been? First, it may have been a direct infection of the cornea with the virus. An instance of the result of direct infection was recorded by Critchett in 1876, in the person of a surgeon who wounded his own eye with the lancet while performing vaccination, thereby contracting a very severe purulent keratitis. Secondly, the keratitis may have been consecutive to a post-vaccinal conjunctivitis. In this case the keratitis, according to Groenouw, can appear under two distinct forms being either an ordinary infiltration or ulcer, situated near the limbus, and healing without much opacity, or a deep keratitis, situated in the centre of the cornea and leaving a dense central macula. Lans thinks the latter form to have been present in his case. The frequency of infection of the eyes by the virus of smallpox has been most favourably influenced by obligatory vaccination. Cohn recorded at the Blind Congress in Breslau in 1901, that before vaccination was made obligatory in Prussia in 1874, 35 per cent. of the blind had lost their eyesight by smallpox. In 1874, in the institutes for blind, only 1 per cent. occurred ; and now-a-days the disease is so rare that the reports of German eye clinics have no column for diseases caused by smallpox.   G. F. ROCHAT.

(17) **Cosmettatos** describes the conditions found in an eye removed on account of a tumour, which started from a papilloma which developed on the site of an old conjunctival wound near the limbus, and after spreading over the entire cornea, began to take on a malignant character. Microscopically, the tumour occupied the anterior part of the cornea, penetrating in the centre almost to Descemet's membrane. It consisted of connective tissue, vessels, and epithelium. The arrangement of the epithelium in places resembled that seen in epithelioma, but from the presence of vessels throughout a large part of the tumour, cither in direct contact with the epithelium or associated with connective tissue, Cosmettatos concludes that the neoplasm was a papilloma tending to undergo epitheliomatous degeneration.

(18) After pointing out that many cases of interstitial keratitis are met with in which no trace of syphilis is observed, **Spicer** has collected 54 cases in which this disease stands out as a distinct clinical entity. Of these 34 occurred in males and 20 in females. The average age of these patients was 40, the oldest being 65 years. Nearly all these patients took alcohol, and many of them took it to excess. Over-eating was clearly present in some cases, and often this was combined with excessive drinking—chiefly of beer. Nine had gout, 7 others rheumatism, and 1 sciatica. Digestive trouble and constipation were present in 7 cases. Carious teeth and pyorrhœa alveolaris were found in 4 cases, and 4 others occurred just before or after the termination of pregnancy. A small number were in perfect health and were abstemious and regular in habits, but had a strong family history of gout. In seven cases the disease seemed to have been started by injury. The average length of the disease was 3 months, and varied from 3 weeks to 12 months. One eye only was affected 27 times, and both eyes 5 times.

Opacification of the cornea either takes the form of a central disc or else of a peripheral cone. In 34 cases "striated keratitis" was present in the early stages, but this very soon disappears, or is hidden by the increasing opacity of the cornea. Œdema of the cornea is nearly always present, and sometimes small bullæ. Fluorescein stains the deeper affected layers at certain stages of the disease, and the endothelium may continue to stain for a long period. Iritis was present in 14 and absent in 34 cases, and the tension was raised in 4 cases. No changes were seen in the fundus, except in one case, where widespread retinal phlebitis appeared after prolonged diarrhœa.

Œdema of the cornea is a marked feature and to this is due the striate keratitis above-mentioned. The deepest fluorescein stained part is due to the shedding of the endothelial cells of Descemet's membrane, which leaves the surface denuded of cells ; this allows the aqueous to infiltrate the deeper layers and thus staining is produced.

It having been proved by Wagenmann, Koster, von Hippel, and others that interference with the blood supply of the ciliary region can experimentally produce parenchymatous keratitis, it is more than likely that the true seat of the disease is an affection of the nutrient blood vessels and that the different forms assumed by the disease are dependent upon the particular vessels affected.

As to treatment, hot fomentations and atropine are the most useful, unless increase of tension precludes use of the latter. Subconjunctival injections of cyanide of mercury or normal saline produce irritation and do no good ; dionine has not proved particularly beneficial. Strict dieting and the treatment of any general condition are of use. Some patients do well with regular doses of mercury, although most of them do equally well without it.   C. D. M.

(19) **Wickerkiewicz's** article deals with certain aspects of that curious affection, Conical Cornea, first clearly described in the year 1748 by Mauchart, of Tübingen, under the name of " staphyloma diaphanum." The condition is usually attributed to diminution in the resistance of the cornea, due to defective innervation, to increased tension, or to feebleness of resistance. The author believes that in conical cornea there is a slight though sensible increase in the intra-ocular tension, and that this, together with a local predisposition connected with nutritional disturbance, brings the condition about. He puts on one side the influence of inflammation (Stellwag) and of endothelial lesions (Panas). With regard to the rhythmical variation in the size of images now and then met with in keratoconus, Wicker- kiewicz has found, by examination with the Javal ophthal- mometer, that it depends upon rhythmical changes in the shape of the apex of the cone. The phenomenon may be unilateral or

bilateral.   He explains the pulsation, after Wagenmann (*Archiv f. Ophthal.*, 44, p. 426), on the analogy of that produced if an aperture leads into a cavity the walls of which contain vascular tissues or fluid, conditions exactly reproduced by an eye with keratoconus.   That the appearance is not invariably present is connected with the fact that the cone is often not thin enough to permit of its production.   Diagnosis, even of commencing conicity, can be made by skiascopy.   With regard to treatment, Wickerkiewicz prefers cauterisation without perforation, whenever the latter can be avoided.   He speaks favourably of Elschnig's modification (*Wiener Klin. Rundschau*, 15 Mai, 1904*).   The author concludes an interesting communication with details of six cases of conical cornea, each of which offers some peculiarity as regards either etiology or progress.   S. S.

(20) Hirschberg reports a case of a girl, *æt.* 9 years, who had marked evidences of tuberculosis, in the shape of ankle joint disease and angular curvature of the spine.   This patient had suffered for two months from a severe inflammation of the left eye, which, on examination under an anæsthetic, was found to present a tumour, resembling granulation tissue, covering the whole of the anterior parts of the eye, and hanging down over the conjunctiva.   A diagnosis of perforating tuberculosis of the iris was made, and the eye consequently enucleated.

Ginsberg, who examined the eye microscopically, found the deeper parts of the eye, including the iris and anterior chamber, quite normal ; Descemet's membrane was intact.   The deeper layers of the cornea were infiltrated with small round cells, and

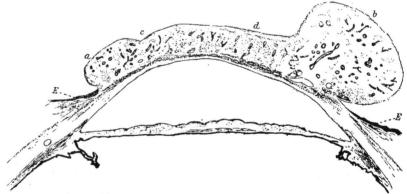

its superficial layers much broken up and in part replaced by this tumour (*see* fig.), which resembled young granulation tissue, and contained many plasma and mast cells.   The tumour might be regarded as a very much exaggerated pannus.   A. Levy.

---

* For abstract see THE OPHTHALMOSCOPE, August, 1904, p. 341.

(21) After mentioning instances of gummata of the cornea published by Magni (1864), Galezowski (1878), Denarié (1882), Lang (1886), and Peters (1898), **Vinsonneau** describes the following case :— a married woman, aged 50 years, has suffered from a gumma of the palate, and a specific paralysis of the right external rectus muscle several years before she fell under the author's notice. There had been one miscarriage. When examined by Vinsonneau, the right cornea was cloudy, except as regards the upper fourth, through which a portion of the iris could be recognised. There were two superficial ulcerations in the cloudy part of the cornea. At the central part of each ulceration lay a clearly - defined figure, of dirty - grey colour, resembling in shape a large comma, and situated in the substance of the cornea. Vision equalled perception of light with the affected eye The diagnosis was made of interstitial keratitis and gummata of the cornea. A gumma of the septum, at the level of the middle meatus, was found in the right nasal fossa. Considerable improvement followed local and general treatment, the latter comprising two series of intramuscular injections of sublimate oil, such as is employed at the Hotêl-Dieu, in Paris, by de Lapersonne.   S. S.

(22) The name keratitis punctata has been applied by different authors to different conditions. Apart from the well-known deposits on Descemet's membrane in cyclitis, there is a kind of interstitial keratitis described by Mauthner and a peculiar form of keratitis made known through Fuchs which go under the same heading. **Jocqs** reports one case of the former and two of the latter description. In a girl, ten years old, numerous yellow-grey irregular specks made their appearance in some part of the cornea, occupying its whole thickness and aecompanied by iritis. Although there was no history or sign of congenital syphilis, mercurial inunction was resorted to, and a cure effected after three months' treatment. In the following two cases of Fuchs's keratitis punctata, which occurred in young male patients, syphilis was more or less evident as the causal agent. The affection is characterised by a rapid onset with photophobia, absence of iritis, and the appearance of a definite number of dots in the anterior layers of the corneal substance. The duration is relatively short (a month or so). The prognosis, therefore, is good.   C. MARKUS.

(23) **Lauber** describes three rare cases of marginal ectasia of the cornea, which, according to his views, differ in several respects from the disease observed by Fuchs (*Archiv f. Ophth.*, LII, 1901, p. 317) and by Terrien (*Archives d'ophtal.*, XX, 1900). Lauber's cases were of chronic inflammatory origin. Material details follow :—(1) A woman, *ætat* 61 years, had remarked for

some years failure of sight in her left eye.   The upper marginal part of the left cornea manifested a semi-lunar, opaque, greyish-white arc, separated by a sharp, irregular line from the rest of the cornea, which had a normal appearance.   The affected part took the form of a shallow groove, the central part of which was ectatic but quite transparent.   Very fine surface vessels covered the affected part.   7 D. of astigmatism.   V.=almost 0·1—6 D. cyl. axis 20°=0·4.   (2) A man, aged 66 years, showed as regards his left eye a finding similar to that described above. The attenuated marginal portion of the cornea lay above and somewhat towards the nasal side, and was bounded below by a sharp line.   Surface vascularisation.   Astigmatism, 13 D. V.+ 1·0 D. sph. with +12 D. cyl. axis 65°=0· 6.   (3) A man, ætat 74 years, had both eyes affected with this peculiar disease. There was slight ectropion of each lower lid, and a markedly hyperæmic conjunctiva.   Pterygium.   Slight mucous discharge. The upper marginal part of each cornea, embracing almost the entire upper half of the cornea, was ectatic, and although traversed by fine superficial vessels, yet retained its transparency. R.V.=2/30 $\frac{-3\cdot0 \text{ sph.}}{-12\cdot0 \text{ cyl. } 40}$·=6/30.   L.V.=3/30, not improved by glasses.   S. S.

(24) There are quite a number of observations which tend to show that diplobacillary conjunctivitis, although usually a slight affection, may be complicated by corneal ulcers. **Paul** describes 26 cases of this kind in which the ulcers were even of a serious type.   The distinctive features of these ulcers consisted in their central situation, an evenly grey or purulent infiltration of the base, the round disc-like shape and the presence of hypopyon and iritis ; the size varied from 2 mm. to 5 mm. in diameter.   A supervening injury was in many instances the immediate cause of the ulcers.   The treatment which Paul found most efficacious, consisted in repeated irrigation with ½% to 1% solution of zinc sulphate, in conjunction with the usual applications in cases of corneal ulceration.   By these means favourable results were, as a rule, attained, although healing was often protracted.

C. Markus.

(25) **Dimmer** describes the case of a man who had several attacks of parenchymatous keratitis, and in whom, several years afterwards, besides the remains of a few vessels, certain grayish markings could be seen in the cornea.   These markings took the form of fine concentric doubly-contoured lines of semi-circular shape and running more or less parallel to the corneal margin ; they were limited to the lower half of the cornea ; and the remains of the blood vessels were in front of them.   These markings were situated in the deepest layers of the cornea.   They are taken by Dimmer to be the effect of folds or wrinkles in the posterior

layers brought about in this case probably by the cornea having swollen during the attack of inflammation and having fallen into folds when returning to its normal condition.   A. LEVY.

(26) **Dimmer** discusses the forms of keratitis described by Fuchs as "keratitis punctata superficialis"; by Adler and v. Reuss as "keratitis maculosa"; and by Stellwag as "keratitis nummularis." These various forms of keratitis have certain well-marked points of difference, and may be regarded as distinct diseases. To them Dimmer now adds a fourth, having certain resemblances to Stellwag's "keratitis nummularis," but also certain points of difference. Thus, there is less conjunctival disturbance than in Stellwag's cases, and the course, which in Stellwag's cases is a rapid one, is very much longer, little change

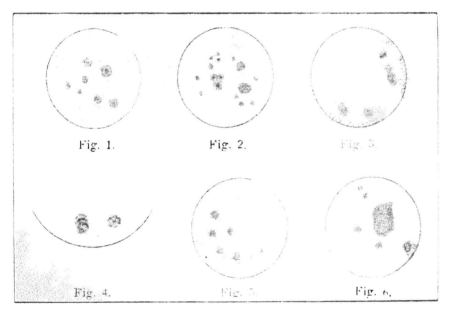

Fig. 1.   Fig. 2.   Fig. 3.

Fig. 4.   Fig. 5.   Fig. 6.

being observed in the course of many weeks' observation. Dimmer's form is that of an infection of the deeper layers of the cornea, in which ulceration is a secondary manifestation occurring late in the disease. Dimmer's drawings are here reproduced. Figs. 1 and 2 represent the right and the left cornea respectively of his first patient, a man aged 63 years. Both conjunctivæ were reddened, but there was no ciliary injection. The infiltrations were small, round spots, 1 mm. to 1.5 mm. in diameter. They had sharp margins of a grey colour, presenting in the centre a small dot or spot of lighter colour. In others, where this spot is not present, the centre is almost transparent. The cornea over them showed fine linear opacities, and a very slight surface depression. The left cornea of this patient was in a similar condition, except that the infiltrations were larger and showed a tendency to confluence. Fig. 3 (with a magnified view in Fig. 4), represents the right cornea of a boy, *ætat* 14 years. The condition came on in the course of three weeks. Here the spots have evidently become confluent, and a few fine vessels are seen. The cornea over them is raised, and in one or two places the epithelium is absent. In the course of a few days, however, these prominences altered into the excavations mentioned above, and the epithelium was regenerated. Three weeks' treatment succeeded in clearing up the condition but slightly.

Fig. 5 represents the right cornea of a man, *ætat* 28 years, whose eye had been injured a month previously by a splash of vinegar. The spots in this case, on careful examination, can be made out to consist of a large number of very fine dots. The cornea over them is raised, with some loss of epithelium. These infiltrations are all in the anterior and middle layers of the cornea. Treatment cleared up the condition but slightly.

Fig. 6 represents the right cornea of a man of 27 years, who three months before got some lime into his eye, an accident, however, from which he recovered perfectly. This cornea has a large number of these infiltrations, some manifestly arising out of the confluence of two or more smaller ones. The largest measures 4 mm. by 3 mm. The larger ones show the denser margin and clearer centre previously noticed, the whole being made up of closely aggregated dots. The condition remained without change in spite of three months' treatment.

Dimmer's cases form, it is obvious, an interesting group, and although none of them has been followed to an end, still their publication is of value, as drawing attention to this curious form of corneal affection. A. LEVY.

(27) **Wehrli** describes two cases in brothers of this interesting affection. He transplanted bits of the nodules into the anterior chamber of guinea pigs, with negative result. Other bits he examined microscopically for tubercle bacilli, and in one section came across two curved vacuolated rods stained red by Ziehl-Nielsen stain, and therefore taken to be tubercle bacilli. He regards the process as analagous to lupus of the skin. He points out the resemblances between these two maladies. A. LEVY.

(28) In **Consiglio's** case an interval of 26 years elapsed between the onset of parenchymatous keratitis in the two eyes. The evidence of hereditary syphilis as the cause of the corneal inflammation, however, is not altogether conclusive. S. S.

(29) **Campbell's** patient, a man, aged 26 years, who exhibited pronounced evidences of hereditary syphilis, was struck in one eye by a flying spark, and a few days later developed typical

interstitial keratitis in the injured eye. The other eye, which had not been injured in any way, became involved about a fortnight later.

(30) **Posey's** patient was a Polish mine labourer, who complained of defective sight. Six months previously the left eye had been struck with a piece of coal, and it had remained inflamed for some time in spite of treatment. About a month after the injury, the right eye also became inflamed ; the inflammation was never very severe, but there was considerable disturbance of vision. The pupillary area of both was the seat of grayish-white opacities of a somewhat oval form ; the epithelium over the opacity was roughened but unbroken ; the opacities extended posteriorly into the *substantia propria* and resolved themselves into a number of grayish clots ; the centre of the opacity was rather denser than the surrounding area. There was no trace of irritation. Subconjunctival saline injections were tried, together with local applications of a 5% solution of iodine and yellow ointment, but the patient eloped from the hospital after two weeks, and was not again seen, so that it is impossible to know whether treatment was of any avail. The literature of this rare disease is given, and, as regards treatment, Fuchs found that atropine, hot compresses, sublimate injections, paracentesis of the anterior chamber, the application of absolute alcohol, etc., were all powerless. The galvano-cautery seems to have cut some cases short, but it entails a scar. Massage should not be used too soon, on account of its liability to excite further irritation.

C. D. M.

(31) **Terson** considers it as proved that gummata of the cornea may occur in syphilis, hereditary or acquired, and that such lesions may be cured, without ulceration, by intensive mercurial treatment, especially by injections of calomel. He describes the following case.—A young woman had suffered from unilateral interstitial keratitis, which was cured in three months. The family and personal evidences of hereditary syphilis were conclusive. Four years after the attack of keratitis, the patient, then aged 22 years, presented a relapse accompanied by violent inflammation of the iris. The limbus and the neighbouring sclera at the lower part of the eye were infiltrated and somewhat swollen, as if the irido-corneal angle were involved. Matters improved for a time under intramuscular injections of mercurial oil, but after twenty injections of the kind had been made, there was a violent relapse of the ocular inflammation. The limbus again became prominent ; two yellowish infiltrations appeared at the lower part of the cornea ; and what Terson and others regarded as a gumma was observed in the external paracentral region of the cornea. The lesion resembled a large tear ; was

clearly defined, and of yellowish colour ; lay in the substance of the cornea, projecting both into the anterior chamber and externally ; and eventually acquired the size of a hemp-seed. Ulceration was not present.   After several injections of calomel, the gumma, although ready to disintegrate, was resorbed, leaving behind it a small opacity only.   H. DE V.

VIII. ATROPHY OF THE IRIS IN TABES AND GENERAL PARALYSIS.

Dupuy-Dutemps.—On a special form of atrophy of the iris in tabes and general paralysis : its relationship to irregularity and reflex disturbances of the pupil.   (Sur une forme spéciale d'atrophie de l'iris au cours du tabes et de la paralysie général : ses rapports avec l'irrégularité et les troubles réflexes de la pupille.) *Annales d'oculistique,* septembre, 1905.

Everybody is aware of the peculiar expression of the eyes in those suffering from tabes dorsalis or general paralysis, an appearance crystallised by Gilles de la Tourette in the brief phrase, " Œil brillant, regard atone." When analysed, this is found to be due to several factors, such as myosis, enophthalmos, narrowing of the palpebral fissure, and the absence of the reaction of the pupil to light. **Dupuy-Dutemps,** however, in the present communica-

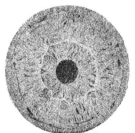   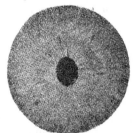

Fig. 1.   Fig. 2.

tion, points to the most important factor of all, namely, modifications in the actual structure of the iris. The normal prominences of the anterior surface (fig. 1), which add not a little to the brilliancy of the iris, are to a large extent in cases presenting the Argyll Robertson pupil, so that the iris becomes flat, as it were, and practically devoid of all relief (fig. 2).   The atrophic changes may involve a portion only of the iris (figs. 3 and 4).   They do not go beyond a certain point, and never attain the extreme degrees observed after serious and prolonged local inflammation.   It is important to note that a precisely similar appearance may be present at a certain stage in the evolution of chronic subacute glaucoma. The atrophic changes are not connected with contraction of the pupil, so often seen in tabes dorsalis. They may even be pronounced in eyes, the pupil of which is large (fig. 4). On the other hand, a distinct relationship exists between the atrophic state of the iris and the deformity of the pupil, which frequently accompanies the Argyll Robertson phenomenon, and, indeed, sometimes

 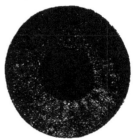

Fig. 3.   Fig. 4

precedes the latter. Thus, the part of the pupillary border which corresponds to the atrophic zone is that which has the greatest radius of curvature. This point may be readily appreciated in figs. 3 and 4, where one sector of the iris is alone involved. The atrophic iris, histologically examined in a single instance, showed a simple atrophy, without signs of inflammatory reaction, involving all the tissues of the iris to an equal extent. The thickness of the stroma was reduced ; while the muscular fibres of the sphincter were united into slender fasciculi, and were less numerous than normal. At certain points pigmentary accumulations were present.

The remainder of this communication is occupied with physiological considerations applied to the explanation of the changes described by Dupuy-Dutemps, but into these highly technical points we have no present intention of entering. For details, readers are referred to the original communication.

S. S.

IX. EXOPHTHALMIC GOITRE.

(1) **Bryant.**—Pigmentation of the eyelids in Graves' disease. *Clinical Journal*, April 26th, 1905.

(2) Teillais.—A new ocular symptom of Basedow's disease. (**Nouveau** symptome oculaire de la maladie de Basedow.) *Archives d'ophtalmologie*, mai, 1905.

(3) **Beaumont, W. M.**—Cases of abnormal eye conditions. *British Medical Journal,* July 8th, 1905.

(1) **Bryant** claims that for many years he has been accustomed to point to pigmentation of the skin of the eyelids as a sign of Graves' disease.

(2) **Teillais,** of Nantes, describes a new and early symptom of Basedow's disease, namely, a brownish pigmentation of the eyelids, sparing the conjunctiva, and ceasing abruptly at the circumference of the orbit.* He narrates three cases in which this abnormal pigmentation was present. The appearance is believed to be related in some way to the known excess of hæmoglobin in the blood of patients affected with exophthalmic goitre.

(3) **Beaumont** reports from the Bath Eye Infirmary cases of—1. Retinitis punctata albescens; 2. Graves's disease; and 3. Essential shrinking of the conjunctiva. The woman suffering from Graves's disease presented a brownish, symmetrical pigmentation of the upper eyelids, in addition to concentric contraction of the field of vision. The latter sign is stated by Beaumont to be not infrequent in that disorder.

REVIEWS.

Transactions of the Ophthalmological Society of the United Kingdom. Volume XXV, 1905. London: J. and A. Churchill, New Burlington Street. Price, 12/6 net.

The *Transactions* of the Ophthalmological Society for 1905 have just made their appearance, and, as usual, represent all that is best as regards the literary side of British ophthalmology. The volume contains 23 plates, numerous diagrams, and upwards of 400 pages of letter-text.

Die lokale Anästhesie in der Augenheilkunde. Von Prof. Dr. BEST, in Giessen. Halle a. S.: Verlag von Carl Marhold. 1905. **Local Anæsthesia in Eye Work.** By Professor BEST, of Giessen. Price, 1 mark 20.

Professor Best's opportune *brochure* deals with the various local anæsthetics that have been and still are used in ophthalmology. After a general discussion of the local and general effects produced by those agents, Best describes, turn by turn, cocaine, acoine, alypin, anæsthesin, chloretone, dionine, eucain β,

* The same symptom, it appears, was described by Schroetter in 1903, and by Jellineck and Rosin in the following year.—EDITORS

holocaine, stövain, subcutin, suprarenin, tropacocaine, and yohimbin. With respect to the latest local anæsthetic, alypin, Best states that the cornea becomes completely anæsthetic within 50 to 75 seconds after a 1% or 2% solution has been applied to the eye. The conjunctiva becomes somewhat hyperæmic, but alypin exerts no action either upon the pupil or the accommodation. The chief advantage of that costly drug, yohimbin, when used as a 0.5% to 1.0% solution, is that the resulting anæsthesia lasts for a long time. Yohimbin produces slight dilatation of the pupil. The booklet concludes with two practical sections— the one dealing with local anæsthesia in operations, and the other as a means for alleviating the pain attending certain diseases of the eye. Cocaine, as well known, mitigates such pain for a short time only, and its continued use under the circumstances is likely to be harmful. Warm applications and the letting of blood are old-fashioned but often efficacious remedies. Radium is too costly for every-day use. As to dionine (nowadays much in vogue as a local analgesic), Best recommends the employment of a 5% solution only as a last resource. It is not altogether clear, however, from his remarks, whether his experiments with that interesting product have gone farther than to apply it to his own eye, naturally with the production of some considerable personal discomfort. S. S.

Colour Vision and Colour Blindness: a Practical Manual for Railroad Surgeons. By J. ELLIS JENNINGS, M.D., St. Louis, Mo., U.S.A. Second Edition. Thoroughly revised with illustrations. 132 pages, crown 8vo. F. A. Davis Company, Publishers, Philadelphia, Pa., U.S.A. Price extra cloth, $1.00 net.

The fact that this book—one upon a special subject in ophthalmology—has passed into its second edition, is sufficient recommendation for its popularity and usefulness. Comparison with the first edition shows careful revision with the introduction of much new matter which is useful. We can heartily endorse the work in every detail; it is one that should be read by every practising ophthalmologist and placed in the hands of every corporation official whose business is to determine colour variations. We believe it to be the best practical manual upon normal and sub-normal colour perception that is now in use. C. A. O.

The Development of the Eye. By J. T. GRADON, M.A. (Oxon.). Leeds: Storey & Co. 1905. Price 3s. 6d.

This book, from which much might be expected by its title, is intended, not for medical students, but for "students of refraction"; it is, in fact, a reprint of articles contributed by the author to the *Dioptric Review*. Only 16 of its 40 pages are taken up by the subject-matter proper, the rest being devoted to contents, preface, and a glossary of embryological terms. An account of the process of karyokinesis is also appended; the striking irrelevancy of this topic only serves to bring into relief the lack of justification that the complication possesses for its existence. The book itself consists of a short summary of the more elementary points relating to the development of the vertebrate eye. There is hardly any of the substance that will not be found in any primer on biology, but the presentation is attractively clear and the style pleasing. From the nature of the monograph but little of the matter calls for any criticism on our part. The writer dogmatically asserts that the views at present accepted, which attribute the origin of the optic nerve to the stalk connecting the fore brain with the optic cup, are quite erroneous; he reserves all discussion of the subject for a further monograph, which we look forward to with interest. He regards the lens capsule as a cuticular membrane deposited by the epithelial cells of the lens and having nothing to do with the mesoblast. The hyaloid membrane he looks on as originating in the same mesoblast as that which forms the vitreous humour. Needless to say, these two last are much disputed topics. In conclusion, we would remark that the diagrams, which are original, are admirable, and constitute the most valuable feature of the book, which is well built throughout. ERNEST JONES.

L'Œil Artificiel. The Artificial Eye. By M. le Docteur ROBERT COULOMB; pp. 152, plates xxvii., and 23 illustrations. Paris: J. B. Baillière et Fils. 1905. Price, 10 francs.

Oculariste is a term for which in English we have no equivalent. Doctor Coulomb is *oculariste* to most of the important ophthalmic hospitals of Paris, and we judge from the present book that an *oculariste* is a maker of artificial eyes. But Dr. Coulomb is no mere artisan, although it is evident he is a very competent artist. He takes a scientific interest in the work he has to do, and the present book is the embodiment of a personal experience evidently of considerable magnitude. It deals with all that is to be known about artificial eyes, and the reading of it would be of value to every ophthalmic surgeon, who usually has to leave himself pretty much in the hands of the mechanician when it comes to having a glass eye fitted for a patient. The operator will find how much can be done in cases where it is seemingly hopeless to get a glass eye fitted, and the photographs show how well a cunning artificer can disguise the presence of the glass eye, even where there is little prothesis left.

Dr. Coulomb discusses very clearly the various methods of removal of the eye, and the methods of dealing with bands, granulations, and contracted sockets. In every respect we regard this little book as well worthy of the attention of ophthalmic surgeons and of *ocularistes* in the British Isles.

LESLIE PATON.

Tratado elemental de Oftalmología. Por el Doctor D. SINFORIANO GARCIA MANSILLA. Madrid: Imprenta y Libreria de Nicolas Moya, Carretas, 8, y Garcilaso, 6. 1905 Price, 20 pesetas. **Elementary Treatise of Ophthalmology.** By Dr. D. SINFORIANO GARCIA MANSILLA, Professor of Ophthalmology in the Faculty of Medicine of Madrid.

This treatise on ophthalmology, the result of much clinical experience in a busy *clinique*, contains 992 pages, 275 illustrations, and two lithographic plates, each including six figures of the fundus and its diseases. It is about the same size as Fuchs's text-book. Dr. Mansilla has arranged the contents of his work under four heads :—1. Anatomy and histology of the visual apparatus ; 2. Physiology ; 3. Methods of examining the eye ; 4. Diseases and pathology. Physiological optics and methods of examination are treated with great clearness. The author has taken considerable pains to study the close relationship that subsists between affections of the eyes and those of the system generally. Dr. Mansilla's treatise, like every book ever written, contains some defects and omissions, but these the author will doubtless correct or supply in later editions. We believe that Dr. Mansilla's book will prove to be the classical Spanish work on ophthalmology. It can be heartily recommended not only to students but also to those practitioners who have already enjoyed some years of practice. E. ALVARADO.

Trachoma. By DR. J. BOLDT, Upper Staff-surgeon and Regimental Surgeon to the 9th West Prussian Infantry Regiment. Translated by J. Herbert Parsons and Thos. Snowball. London : Hodder & Stoughton, 1904, pp. 232. Price 7s. 6d. *net.*

Alien immigration has been responsible lately for several things, among them for the present translation of Dr. J. Boldt's *Trachom als Volks-und HeeresKrankheit*, 1903. Messrs. J. H. Parsons and Thomas Snowball have done the work of translation in a scholarly way, and have managed to produce a tolerably readable volume from somewhat unpromising material. The book, however, is stuffed with statistics, and resembles nothing so much as a cyclopædia. It deals with the history, epidemiology, distribution, symptoms, course, ætiology, diagnosis, prognosis, treatment, and prophylaxis of trachoma, and it is pretty safe to say that few aspects of that disease are neglected. At the same time, the book contains nothing in the least original, and nothing that could not have been produced by an intelligent individual possessed of the necessary perseverance and having access to a well-equipped medical library. In a sense it may be said to recall Sattler's famous *Die Trachombehandlung einst und jetzt* (1891), although without having the practical aim and personal note that formed such distinctive features in the latter production. In view of these facts, it becomes a little difficult to comprehend the reasons that have led to the publication of the present English translation. The book abounds, as might be expected, with references to German, Austrian, Belgian, and French literature. That English literature, on the other hand, is somewhat of a *terra incognita* to the learned and laborious author, will be apparent from the bald fact that the extensive bibliography contains no allusion to the names of Shuttleworth, Mowat, Nettleship, Bridges, Litteljohn, Stephenson, Hutchinson, and others, who in England have written upon the subject of trachoma. Of the earlier British writers, Vetch (1817) is the only one that figures in Dr. Boldt's list. The splendid work of Saunders (1811), Farrell (1811), Ware (1808-1814), MacGregor (1812), Edmonston (1824), O'Halloran (1824), Frank (1860), Weleh (1860), and Marston (1862), is passed over without a mention of their names in the bibliography. Yet our present-day knowledge of ophthalmia is owing, in no small measure, to the brilliant researches made in the nineteenth century by these and by other workers.

This omission probably accounts for the somewhat anomalous fact that an introductory chapter, dealing with trachoma in the British Isles, has been contributed to the volume by Mr. E. T. Collins. It must be confessed that, to our mind, Mr. Collins' forty-two pages are of more value than all the rest of the book put together. They provide us with a concise and clearly-written account of epidemic trachoma in Britain and her over-sea dependencies from the return of Sir Ralph Abercromby's troops in 1801 and the following year to the present day. The destructive ophthalmia of the earlier part of the nineteenth century was probably partly gonorrhœal and partly trachomatous. Mr. Collins surmises that the attenuated disease, as it prevails to-day, is due to the absence of the gonorrhœal element, to which he might have added, as potent contributory factors, the great all-round improvement in sanitary conditions, the care that is now taken with epidemic ophthalmia at the outset, and, last but not least, improved methods both of prevention and of treatment. The course of trachoma in the British Army is traced by Mr. Collins, and in this connection it is interesting to note that, by the military authorities, the extermination of the scourge is attributed to every soldier having a towel of his own, to the unlimited supply of water, and to the better ventilation of the barracks occupied by the men. Mr. Collins then passes forward to describe what may be conveniently called the " ophthalmic history " of the London Poor-Law Schools, of which the first was opened in the year 1849 at Norwood, in Surrey. Some of the more important outbreaks of epidemic ophthalmia that have broken out in these schools are touched upon. The establishment in 1889 of the Ophthalmic School at Hanwell, in order to cope with such an outbreak in the Central District School, is mentioned, and the details that led to its being thrown open to the metropolis in 1893 are alluded to. Lastly, Mr. Collins outlines the steps whereby the Metropolitan Asylums Board were eventually constituted the authority responsible for trachoma cases among the infantile poor-law population. The Asylums Board, as well known, has built two schools for treatment of the disease, one at Brentwood and the other at Swanley. The arrangements, structural and domestic, of these two costly institutions are described, and some idea is given by Mr. Collins of the way the work is carried on. Incidentally mention is made of the modern treatment of trachoma by X-rays and radium, and from this account it appears that the former agent has yielded satisfactory results. Finally, Mr. Collins directs attention to aliens and their influence as a source of trachoma in this country ; but into this somewhat vexed question, about which there is yet much to be learned, we have no present intention of entering.

Die Wirkungen von Arzneimitteln und Giften auf das Auge. Handbuch für die gesammte ärztliche Praxis. Von Dr. L. LEWIN, Professor in Berlin, und Dr. H. GUILLERY, Professor in Cöln. In zwei Bände, mit 99 Textfiguren. Berlin : Hirschwald, 1905, pp. 857 und 1044. **The Action of Drugs and Poisons on the Eye** : A Manual for general medical practice, by Dr. L. LEWIN, Professor in Berlin, and Dr. H. GUILLERY, Professor in Cologne. 1905. Price 52 M.
Professor Lewin and Guillery's work is very useful and welcome. It is the first attempt to supply a complete account of the pharmacology and toxic agents affecting the eye. Numerous drugs have been prescribed in the treatment of diseases of the eye, and excellent papers have been written giving an account of the action of the chief remedies, but these are distributed through *Transactions* of learned societies or lie buried in journals, only to be discovered after long and

wearisome search in their pages or indices. It is, therefore, with great pleasure that in these handsome volumes we find the scattered facts collected, and a reliable account given, not only of the various drugs that have been employed, but of those noxious agents which have been found to impair or to destroy the function of sight, whether taken internally, as in the case of alcohol and tobacco, or topically applied, as in that of the various micro-organisms, and the large group of chemical and physiologically active substances. Many of the latter here described are un-known even to well-informed practitioners, such, for example, as atroscin, mydrol, lactyl tropin, tropyl-lupinin, peronin, and others ; short distinctive trade names having been found imperative in view of the extraordinarily complex constitution which some of them possess ; nirvanin, for example, which is an uncertain local anæsthetic, being represented by the appalling chemical name of diethylglycocoll-amido-oxybenzoicacidmethyl ester.

The general arrangement of the work is that the first volume is occupied with the consideration (1) of those substances which exert a paralysing influence on the nervous system ; (2) of those which stimulate or excite the nervous system, and, lastly, (3) of those substances which exert a chemical or physical action upon the metabolism of living proteids. The second volume is almost exclusively taken up with the action of the different forms of bacteria, and with the action of local irritants and poisons. The first of these sections includes chloroform, ether, opium and its derivatives, and local anæsthetics and mydriatics. The second includes alcohol and ethereal oils, tobacco, strychnia, coffee, tea, and local myotics. The third embraces the metalloids and metals, metabolic poisons, like the ptomaines and toxins, which lead to cataract, whilst in the second volume the reader will find a *résumé* of all that is known in regard to the action of the gonococcus, staphylococcus, streptococcus, pneumococcus, and the bacillus tuberculosis, which last is discussed at great length and very instructively. Throughout both volumes illus-trative cases, drawn from the works of writers of repute, are given and add greatly to the value of the statements made, as well as to the opinions held by the authors themselves. In many instances the action of drugs upon animals is given, as well as on man. Thus, in regard to one important drug, physostigmine, it is stated that the action in various animals is different, cats and dogs responding strongly, whilst in the rabbit, in amphibia, and fish the myotic effect is slight or imperceptible. In the cat, a drop of a one-half per cent. solution causes very pronounced myosis, though the pupillary borders do not completely meet. In pigeons very small doses cause oscillation of the pupil with a tendency to contraction, but larger ones reduce the size of the pupil to 1·5 mm. In man the extract of calabar bean produces constriction of the pupil in from 8 to 15 minutes, the effects lasting from two to three days. The weakest solution of physostigmine which perceptibly acts on the pupil is 1 in 12,800 parts of water. The times of action of 0·5 and of 1 and 2 per cent. of physostigmine are given. Maximum contraction with 2 per cent. solutions, is established in from 15 to 20 minutes. A full account is then given of the effects of this agent on the accommodation, some of the authorities quoted being v. Reuss, Mohr, Königstein, Zehender, Jaarsma, Donders, Krenchel, Hess, Lang and Barrett. To this succeeds a description of the imbalance, or want of balance, of the muscles of the eye caused by eserin, the disturbances of vision caused by the change in the diameter of the pupil and the alteration of the accommodation ; the changes that may be seen in the fundus of the eye ; the changes in the intra-ocular pressure ; the effects of the drug on the limits of the field ; impairment of the acuteness of vision and its effects in producing nystagmus and spasm of the orbicularis ; disturbance of the conjunctiva and of the parts surrounding the globe; lastly, the general symptoms produced by an overdose of the poison.

The section on the metalloids, metals, and acids, embraces the following subjects : iodine, and its preparations ; arsenic ; phosphorus ; mercury ; bismuth ; chromium ; lead ; antimony; and sulphuric acid. Of these, the chapter on lead may be selected as constituting a monograph of great value. It extends to over a hundred pages, and gives full details of cases, derived from many sources, of the optic neuritis observed in lead poisoning and its terminations in recovery, atrophy, or death ; of albuminuric retinitis with or without albuminuria ; hemianopsia and disturbances of the function of the ocular muscles ; of the ætiology of saturnine amaurosis, and, finally, of the local toxic effects of lead on the conjunctiva.

There is also a full account of the effects of animal poisons, commencing with the hairs of certain caterpillars, the effects of which are often very serious, such as is seen in those of the Gastropacha pini, rubi, trifolii, and quercifolia ; those of Bombyx rubi, and lanestris ; of Cnethocampa processionæ ; of Lasiocampa potatoria, pini, and quercifolia ; of Liparis monacha ; Arctia caja; Pieris brassica, Portesia chrysorrhœa and auriflua and of Morpho metellus, in all of which the hairs appear to be poisonous to man, and even animals do not appear to be immune, since they present in many instances the same local and general effects, and quit woods where such caterpillars abound. The inflammation excited is divided into two chief forms, Erucismus inflammatorius and Erucismus nodulosus, in accordance with the symptoms produced. Treatment has not proved very efficacious, but weak carbonate

THE OPHTHALMOSCOPE.

of soda solutions and the application of parsley seem to be the best means. Other animal poisons are those of bees, wasps, ants, spiders, the centipede and scorpion, with a list of Diptera, too long to quote, and there is a long list also of Epizoa and Entozoa, which have been found at different times in or on the eye.

HENRY POWER.

(*To be concluded.*)

NOTES AND ECHOES.

British Medical Association. THE British Medical Association, as readers need scarcely be reminded, will hold its annual gathering in August, 1906, at Toronto, Canada. The local branch of the Association has paid a high compliment to ophthalmology in nominating for the office of President Dr. R. A. Reeve. Dr. Reeve, in addition to holding several other dignified appointments, is professor of ophthalmology and otology in the University of Toronto. THE OPHTHALMOSCOPE congratulates both Dr. Reeve and the Association upon the appointment.

*   *   *   *

Obituary. FROM Montreal the death is announced, at the age of 61 years, of Dr. Frank Buller,* at one time house-surgeon to the Moorfields Hospital, London. He introduced the well-known watch-glass and sticking-plaster shield that goes by his name. Buller graduated in 1869 from Victoria University, Coburg, Ontario, and for seventeen years held the post of ophthalmologist and aurist to the Montreal General Hospital. A few years ago he accepted a similar position on the staff of the Royal Victoria Hospital. Since the year 1883 Buller has been professor of ophthalmology in McGill University. He was a member of the Ophthalmological Society of the United Kingdom. The deaths are also announced of Dr. Louis J. A. Simard, oculist, of Quebec City, and of Dr. J. O. Brookhouse, one of the founders of the Nottingham and Midland Eye Infirmary.

*   *   *   *

News Items. THE Congress for the Repression of the illegal Practice of Medicine, will meet in Paris, under the presidency of Professor Brouardel, on the 30th April, 1906. Dr. Péchin, of Paris, will open a discussion on the

The next number of THE OPHTHALMOSCOPE will contain a biographical sketch of Buller. written by his intimate friend, Dr. J. Gardner, of Montreal, Canada.— EDITORS.

illegal exercise of ophthalmology. A very practical step has been taken by the Chicago, Milwaukee, and St. Paul Railroad. The men employed by that line complain that their eyes are tested on theoretical rather than on practical grounds. The management have therefore arranged to place ophthalmic surgeons on the engines drawing the express trains, in order to make tests and to examine the exact conditions under which train signals are displayed. The whole question of sight and colour testing will be revised in the light of the knowledge obtained in this way. Arthur H. H. Sinclair, M.D., F.R.C.S.E., has been appointed, for a term of five years, assistant ophthalmic surgeon to the Edinburgh Royal Infirmary. The following gentlemen have been nominated examiners for 1905-1906 in ophthalmic surgery for the diploma of the Fellowship of the Royal College of Surgeons of Edinburgh : George A. Berry, George Mackay, William George Sym, and James Veitch Paterson. Dr. E. Moreau has been appointed *chef de clinique* in the ophthalmological service of service of Professor E. Rollet, at Lyon, France. Legacies have accrued to the Tunbridge Wells Eye Hospital and to the Norfolk and Norwich Eye Hospital.

*　　　*　　　*　　　*

Ophthalmological Society. THE 1905-1906 session of the Ophthalmological Society was inaugurated on October 19th, when the new President, Mr. Priestley Smith, delivered an address on the changes of method in ophthalmology that he had experienced during the last quarter of a century. As exemplified by himself, he traced the gradual evolution and widening of an eye specialist, who to begin with, paid scant attention to the importance of general methods, and later began to see things in their true perspective. In a word, Mr. Priestley Smith dwelt upon the importance of environment and personal habits. The influence of alcohol, tobacco, diet, holidays, and a thousand and one things of that description were touched upon by the lecturer in a more or less interesting way.

*　　　*　　　*　　　*

London Medical Societies: Amalgamation Scheme. SPEAKING of medical societies brings one by a process of easy transition to the burning question that is now agitating most of the London medical societies, namely, the amalgamation scheme promoted and fostered by the Royal Medical and Chirurgical Society. A report has recently been issued by the Executive Committee, with regard to this important question of fusion. The 22 societies named in the report as suitable for fusion into an Academy of Medicine would undoubtedly form a large, and in some respects a powerful, organisation. Looking at the scheme from a financial

point of view, the figures given by the Committee do not allow
of a large balance of income over expenditure. If the new body
is to be a success, it must not be crippled financially. The
estimate given appears to provide for bare necessities only, and
does not allow for the many items of expenditure which in the
event of amalgamation will be sure to turn up in the initial stage.
The large debenture debt, over £33,000, of the Royal Medical
and Chirurgical Society is unfortunate, as is also the fact that the
income (£436) from the Berners Street property ceased at the
end of 1904. This considerably weakens the financial position,
for a larger sum will have to be provided annually to pay interest
alone. With regard to the societies possessing properties and
funds, how are they going to benefit by amalgamation? Take
the Society in which many of our readers are interested,
the Ophthalmological. At the present time the members pay
£1 1s. 0d. per annum, which entitles them to all the benefits of the
Society, including the privilege of attending all meetings, the
volume of *Transactions*, and, last but not least, the use of the fine
special library. If the new Society materialize (which is doubtful)
and the Ophthalmological Society decide to join (which is, to
say the least of it, still more doubtful), the members will
have to pay one guinea to join, and a second guinea if they
want to use the library, In other words, they will have to pay
two guineas for what now costs them one guinea. But that is
not the worst, for under the scheme outlined by the committee,
the members of the Ophthalmological Section would lose the
power of electing the members of their own special section, inasmuch as the power of veto is vested in the hands of the Council
of the Academy of Medicine ; male and female members would be
eligible for election ; and the individual interest now taken by men
in such a society as the Ophthalmological would probably dwindle
away when the society was merged in the Academy of Medicine.
The majority of the smaller societies appear to be doing good
and useful work, by building up libraries, arranging lectures and
clinical meetings, publishing *Transactions*, and, in many cases
accumulating funds, which, if need be, could be utilised for
special research work. The Academy, if it come into existence,
purposes to take all libraries and all the invested funds of the
respective societies, so that the strong will have to help the weak.
But it does not at all appear that this assistance will be sufficient
to maintain such a society as is proposed by the committee. It
was said at the meeting at the College of Physicians earlier in
the year that the various societies, as at present constituted,
would lose their individuality. The result will be that members
of sections will be liable to lose to some extent their interest,
because it is a very different thing to be a member of a section

and a member of a self-contained society, managed without any control from a higher authority. At present the members of the smaller societies feel that they can take some part in the management of affairs, and they may aspire to hold office in such societies. This interest spells success from every point of view. It is doubtful if such interest would be taken in a mere section of a large society. The distinction between a " Fellow " and a " Member " of the Academy is at present the mere difference between £3 3s. od., and £1 1s. od., per annum, and a distinctly tempting bait is held out to certain men when they learn that at first, provided only they belong to any of the 22 societies named in the schedule, they can become " Fellows " of the Academy of Medicine without ballot and without entrance fee. It may be noticed that several of the societies included in the scheme already have lady members such as the Obstetrical, the Society of Anæsthetists, the Medico-Psychological, and possibly others. Indeed, there are many details in the scheme proposed by the committee that lie open to serious and possibly to destructive criticism.

*   *   *   *

Ophthalmology in Japan. A RECENT number (October, 1905) of Dr. Würdemann's excellent periodical, *Ophthalmology*, contains some interesting details concerning eye work in "the land of the rising sun." Ume, Suda, and Tatsuya Inouye are credited with having created modern ophthalmology in Japan. Japan now has three medical faculties (Tokio, Kyoto, and Fuknoka), one higher medical school (Osaka), and nine general medical schools. These various institutions have eleven professors of ophthalmology. Most of the twenty-nine eye specialists have studied in Germany. There is one journal devoted to ophthalmology, the *Nippon-Gankwa-Gakkwai-Zasshi*, published by Professor Onishi in Fuknoka.

*   *   *   *

Ophthalmology in France. CONTRAST with this the conditions in France. The October number of our contemporary, *L'Ophtalmologie Provinciale*, contains quite a pathetic account by Dr. Bourgeois of his failure to establish a chair of ophthalmology at Rheims, an important town of 108,000 inhabitants. The general hospital at that place appears to possess no special eye department! Dr. Bourgeois tells us that he prefers to operate upon indigent patients at his private *clinique* rather than at the hospital, where the lighting is bad, and eye cases are scattered about among the general surgical beds. In 1902 Bourgeois obtained the permission of the authorities to hold a course of lectures on elementary ophthalmology, consisting of about twelve lectures, during the summer session.   Ten students availed themselves of the privilege.   But during the next year a change had come over the spirit of the dream, inasmuch as the students seemed to resent this addition to their existing burdens.   Bourgeois accordingly suggested that the course should be made obligatory, and be included among the other clinical lectures given to the students.   His suggestion, however, that a chair of ophthalmology should be founded, was negatived by the powers that be.   Upon this refusal on the part of the authorities, Bourgeois abandoned his fixed lectures, although at the same time he has announced that students will be welcomed at his *clinique*.   He now demands that a chair of clinical ophthalmology at each medical school shall be proposed by the Minister of Public Instruction and decreed by the President of the French Republic. It appears that, as matters stand, there are two professors of ophthalmology only among about a dozen of the French provincial schools of medicine, namely, at Angers and at Lyon.

*   *   *

A Study in Bibliography.   IN a letter in a recent issue of the *Ophthalmic Record* Dr. Edward Jackson, of Denver, U.S.A., has aired a grievance.   It seems that in reviewing that useful compilation the "Ophthalmic Year Book" the *Centralblatt für praktische Augenheilkunde*, adopted the somewhat unusual course of selecting, apparently at random, half a dozen authors and of contrasting by means of "the deadly parallel," the references to their writings as given in the "Year Book" and in the corresponding volume of the *Centralblatt*.   The comparison turned naturally in favour of the last-named publication. Dr. Jackson, with a fine touch of irony, looked up the references in the *Centralblatt*, as he says, " hoping to find in what directions the Year Book was most defective."   The result was distinctly amusing.   The Year Book covered the literature for 1903, while the *Centralblatt.* including its supplement (which appeared several months after the close of the year) was supposed to cover a similar period.   Dr. Jackson found that of the three references in the *Centralblatt* to papers by Fuchs, two were published in 1902, and the third was mentioned in the Year Book.   Of the eight references to Cirincione, as given in the *Centralblatt*, two belonged to 1902, one was in the nature of a controversial letter, a third was a duplicate reference to an article that had been published in two journals, while five references were given in both periodicals.   And so on for the other writers selected for this unhappy and invidious comparison.

Dr. Jackson, however, does not rest content with this explanation, but being evidently a born controversialist, carries the war
into the enemy's camp. Leaving on one side European
writers, he sets out to enquire how the *Centralblatt* had dealt
with American authors, and gives the following figures :—

	Year Book.	Centralblatt.
A. Duane	6 ...	3
Friedenberg	5 ...	1
F. C. Hotz	3 ...	1
C. R. Holmes	1 ...	0
A. Knapp	3 ...	0
G. M. Gould	5 ...	0

Dr. Jackson points out that of the 164 American authors referred
to in the Year Book, 64 were not mentioned in the *Centralblatt*.
He concludes his letter with the following parting shot :—
" In the way of suggesting improved methods for bibliographic
work, this study of German thoroughness was disappointing ; but it
was rather soothing to one who felt regret for the shortcomings
of the Year Book."

Edinburgh Royal Infirmary. AT a recent meeting of the Managers of the
Edinburgh Royal Infirmary the following
minute was adopted with regard to the
retirement of the senior ophthalmic surgeon :—

" The Managers regret that, in consequence of the expiry of his term of
office, they must lose the services of Mr. George A. Berry as Senior Surgeon in
the Eye Department. They desire to convey to him their sincere thanks for the
able and untiring service which he has given the institution during the long
period of twenty-three years. They are grateful that a man possessing a world-
wide reputation, because of his ability in his special department of surgery, has
devoted so much time to the gratuitous care of the afflicted poor. They hope
that Mr. Berry's extensive knowledge, operative ability, and other talents may
continue to receive that public confidence and recognition which they so richly
deserve. In token of their esteem and of their appreciation of his work, the
Managers appoint him one of the consulting surgeons to the Eye Department of
the Institution."

*

University College, Bristol. THE prospectus for 1905-1906 of University
College, Bristol, which, be it remembered
possesses a medical school of some impor-
tance, is adorned with an advertisement of a firm of " eyesight
and spectacle specialists," recommending students to consult
them at their "eyesight testing rooms." *Que diable allait-il
dans cette galère ?*

TO SUBSCRIBERS AND CONTRIBUTORS.

Cloth Cases for binding Vol. II. are now ready and can be obtained upon application to the Publishers.   Price 2/-.

Subscribers living in the United Kingdom should receive their copies on the 1st of every month, and it is requested that any delay in delivery may at once be communicated to the London Office.

For the information of subscribers in the British Colonies, United States, &c., it may be stated that *The Ophthalmoscope* is posted in London on the last day of the month preceding the date borne by the journal.

Terms, including postage, payable in advance, 10s. 6d. (2 dollars and 56 cents) for 12 months.   Single copies 1s. (25 cents).

All remittances should be made payable to the "Manager of *The Ophthalmoscope*" at 24, Thayer Street, London, W., England, except American remittances, which should be addressed to the office of the American Editor, 1507, Locust Street, Philadelphia, U.S.A.

Reprints of articles appearing in *The Ophthalmoscope* can be obtained at reduced rates, provided application be made before the type is distributed ; notification of such should be placed upon the original copy, or sent when returning corrected proofs.

Reprints may be obtained at the following rates :—

	s. d.		s. d.		s. d.
25 copies of 4 pp.	5 6	Of 8 pp.	8 6	Extra for covers	4 0
50 ,, ,,	6 6	,,	10 0	,,	5 0
100 ,, ,,	8 6	,,	14 0	..	6 6
200 ,, ,,	12 6	,,	21 0	,,	9 0

Original contributions, books for review, material for abstract purposes, news items, etc., from America, are to be sent to 1507, Locust Street, Philadelphia, U.S.A. ; those from Great Britain and all other countries to 24-26, Thayer Street, London, W., England.

Applications for reprints are to be made to the "Manager of *The Ophthalmoscope*," 24-26, Thayer Street, London. England, or to the American Editor, 1507, Locust Street, Philadelphia U.S.A.

Applications for Advertisements to be made to :—
THE MANAGER OF "THE OPHTHALMOSCOPE," 24-26, THAYER STREET, LONDON.

ADVERTISEMENTS. V.

[NOW READY, Price 3s. net.]

HE BLIND MAN'S WORLD,

English version of ENTRE AVEUGLES: Advice to people who have recently lost
r sight, by DR. ÉMILE JAVAL, Directeur Honoraire du Laboratoire d'Ophtalmologie de
cole des Hautes Études; Membre de l'Académie de Médecine. Translated by ERNEST
OMSON, M A., M.D., Fellow of the Faculty of Physicians and Surgeons of Glasgow, Surgeon
he Glasgow Eye Infirmary, Ophthalmic Surgeon Glasgow Maternity Hospital, formerly
fessor of Physiology in Anderson's College Medical School. etc.

PRESS NOTICES.

"This is the translation of an important w rk which should be in the hands of those who
have the comfort and well being of the blind entrusted to them. . . . We strongly recom-
mend this book to all those who have the care of the blind; those who have had the
misfortune to lose the priceless blessing of vision can learn much from it, if it be read to them
by a sympathetic companion."—*Lancet*.

"For those whom Dr. Javal has in view his book is a treasury of consolatory stimulation.
and it will encourage them to hold their own unt.l they subdue and override the tyranny of
darkness."—*Sheffield Telegraph*.

"It deserves the wider circulation which Dr. Ernest Thomson's admirable English version
will secu e for it. and it may be read with profit as well as interest, not only by the friends of
the blind, but by the general public. . . . This most interesting book contains a mine of
information as to the doings of the blind, which is bound to be specially helpful and suggestive
to all who have the happiness of this class at heart." *Glasgow Herald*.

"The book will prove a comfort and an inspiration to many a sightless pessimist."—
Dundee Advertiser.

"The book contains many hints which will be most useful to those on whom the terrible
affliction of blindness has fallen."—*Belfast News-Letter*.

"That the work is one which everyone should read, both for pleasure and profit, is the
least that can be said of this book, which has been actually written by a blind man. The
work of the translator has been faithfully performed.'—*Medical Press and Circular*.

ONDON: GEORGE PULMAN & SONS, THAYER STREET, W.

JOHN L. BORSCH'S PATENT
KRYPTOK is the only
Invisible Bifocal Lens.

Awarded the
OLD MEDAL
at the
LOUISIANA
PURCHASE
EXPOSITION.

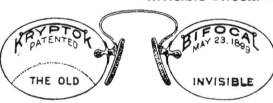

Neat, Durable,
Perfect.

Enjoys the Highest
Endorsements.

Patented in Europe, and the United States of America. WRITE FOR FREE BOOKLET.

OHN L. BORSCH & Co., Manufacturing Opticians,

1324, Walnut Street, 217, So. Ninth Street, PHILADELPHIA, P.A., U.S.A.

By A. H. TUBBY, M.S.

DEFORMITIES: A TREATISE ON ORTHOPÆDIC SURGERY.
Six hundred pages. Three hundred Illustrations. PRICE 17s.
BRIT. MED JOURNAL.—"Standard work on the subject in the English language.'
London: MACMILLAN & CO., LTD., St. Martin's Street, W.C.

APPENDICITIS. Ninety-two pages. PRICE 2s 6d.
BRIT. MED. JOURNAL.—"Reviews lucidly and instructively the main points of the affection.
London: BAILLIERE, TINDALL & COX, 8, Henrietta Street, Strand, W.C.

CLINICAL LECTURES ON INTRA-ABDOMINAL SUPPURATION.
One hundred and four pages. PRICE 3s 6d.
BRIT. MED. JOURNAL.—"Will prove useful to those who wish for a concise clinical account of the various forms.
London: THE MEDICAL PUBLISHING COMPANY, LTD., 22½. Bartholomew Close, E.C.

**THE PREVENTIVE AND CURATIVE TREATMENT OF ENLARGED GLANDS
OF THE NECK.** PRICE 1s
London: THE MEDICAL PUBLISHING COMPANY, LTD., 22½, Bartholomew Close, E.C·

vi. ADVERTISEMENTS.

ARTHUR W. HEAD, F.Z.S

OPHTHALMIC ARTIST,

26, DORNTON ROAD, BALHAM, S.W.

Drawings in black and white, or in colours, made of all ocular conditions, external and inter

OPTICAL LANTERN SLIDES a Speciality.

ARTIFICIAL EYES.

WILLIAM HALFORD, Senr.,

Practical Maker,

41, UPPER TOLLINGTON PARK, N.,

And 104, MARYLEBONE ROAD,

(By Special Appointment to the Royal London Ophthalmic Hospital, City Road, E.C.)

REFORM AND ORDINARY SHELL EYES ACCURATELY FITTE

MARTINDALE'S
STERILIZED DRESSINGS.

Specially suitable for the requirements of Ophthalmic Surgeons.

We guarantee these Dressings have been submitted to a temperature of 250° F, for 30 minutes at a pres
of 15 lbs. in a steam vacuum autoclave, after the methods of Pasteur and Lister.

Before sterilization each parcel of Dressing is completely enveloped in a sheet of cotton wool, which
is well-known, constitutes the most perfect method for the exclusion of bacteria. The wool wrapping rem
on, and is only removed the moment the surgeon requires the Dressing. As a further precaution, each pa
is wrapped in parchment paper, and placed in an air-tight, dust-proof carton.

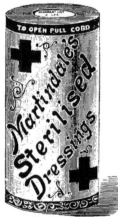

		Absorbent. Per doz. Cartons.		Alembroth. Per doz. Cartons.		Boric. Per doz. Cartons.		Cyanid Per doz. Cartons.
Gauze	1 yard 5/-		..	6/-	...	6/-	...	6/6
,,	2 yards 8/6			10/-	...	10/6	...	12/-
,,	6 ,, 18/-			—	...	—	...	24/-
,,	12 ,, —		...	—	...	—	...	36/-
Lint	1 oz. 5/-		..	6,-	...	5/6	...	7/-
,,	2 ozs. 9/-		...	9/-	...	8/-	...	10/-
Swabs	6 in carton (Plain Absorbent)		...	per doz. cartons 12/-				
,,	smaller size, 12 in carton (Plain Absorbent)							
	especially suitable for eye work					,,	...	9/-
Wool	1 oz. 4/-		...	5/6	...	5/3	...	7/-
,,	2 ozs 5/9		...	7/6	...	7/-	...	10/-
,,	8 ozs. 13/-		...	—	...	—	...	—

In addition are packed Bandages, Wrappers, Towels, etc. Full list on
application.

W. MARTINDALE,

Manufacturing & Analytical Chemis

10, NEW CAVENDISH STREET, LONDON, W.

We hold largest stock in London of new preparations, and are in a positi
to supply the same on favourable terms, *vide* Monthly List. Post orders a
specially attended to, and promptness in despatch is guaranteed.

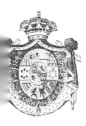 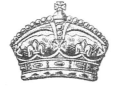 

Established 1750.

Dollond & Co.,

**Spectacle
Manufacturers &
Lens Grinders.**

Opticians

To Members of the British and Danish Royal Families.
The Empress of Russia, The King of Spain, etc.

Messrs. Dollond & Co. beg to introduce to the notice of
the Medical Profession their wonderful new lenses for
Spectacles:

ISOMETROPE LENSES.

Obtain clearer vision
with less fatigue.

10 per cent. less
curvature (for equal
focus) than ordinary
glasses.

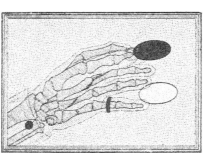

TRADE MARK.

They entirely
eliminate and prevent
the ultra-violet and
other harmful rays
from entering the eyes.

They have great
advantages over all
other spectacle lenses
on the market.

Descriptive booklet containing reports of many eminent authorities post free on application.

DOLLOND & Co., 35, Ludgate Hill, E.C.

BRANCHES:

223, Oxford Street, W.   113, Cheapside, E.C.
5, Northumberland Avenue, Charing Cross, W.C.
Next to First Avenue Hotel, High Holborn.
62, Old Broad Street, E.C.

Free demonstrations with x-ray apparatus, &c., all day at 113, Cheapside, E.C.

Personal enquiries and correspondence are cordially invited.

viii.   ADVERTISEMENTS

Telephone: 9362 CENTRAL.

Worth's Amblyoscope

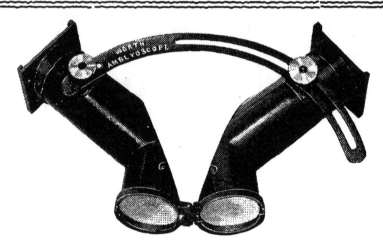

A. HAWES, Established 1840

Prescription Optician,

79, Leadenhall Street, E.C
AND . .
49, New Cavendish St., W

Optician to Royal London Ophthalmic Hospital, City Road, E.C
and London Hospital, E., &c.

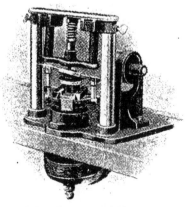

MACHINE USED FOR WORKING TOROIDAL
LENSES.

Cases of Trial Test Lenses, any size a
description, made to order.

"MOORFIELDS" ADJUSTABLE TRI
FRAMES.

Test Types, Retinoscopy, Mirrors, etc., e

MARINE, FIELD, and OPERA GLASSI

Toroidal, Cylindrical, and other Len
carefully worked to prescription.

ADVERTISEMENTS.

ESTABLISHED 1777.

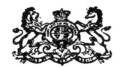

TO H.M. THE KING.   TO H.M. THE QUEEN.

C. W. DIXEY & SON,

MANUFACTURING OPTICIANS,

3, NEW BOND STREET, LONDON, W.

AND 20, WELBECK STREET, W.

(No other address.)

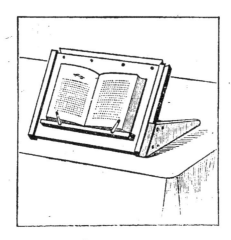

The Englefield Book-Support ensures a correct position in reading.
should be useful to all, but especially to children who wear spectacles.
reduces the *difference* of distance between the top and bottom of the
ge of a book, ensures an upright position for the head, and avoids oblique
ght through the margin of the spectacle lens.

Prices :

In canary wood, 12 in. by 16 in. 5/-
Do.   stained and polished   ...   6/-
In oak, plain, 6/6 ;   polished, 7/6.

The Book-Support may be seen at the Bond Street or Welbeck Street
ops ;   or a sample will be sent on receipt of a request.

GEORGE SPILLER

Surgeons' Optician,

3, WIGMORE STREET

LONDON, W.

Telephone: 636, MAYFAIR.

IN COURSE OF PREPARATION—

A NEW FRAMELESS PINCE-NEZ:

The "Spillerflex.

(Patent No. 14637, 1905.   Foreign Patents applied for.)

No Holes.   No Screws.
Lenses cannot rock

A COMBINATION OF NEATNESS, DURABILITY, AND OPTIC
ACCURACY.

CPSIA information can be obtained
at www.ICGtesting.com
Printed in the USA
BVHW091310210219
540827BV00022B/1757/P

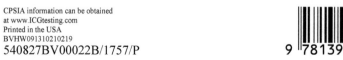